Shredding Suicide's Lie

There Is Another Way

Linda Arbizu

LFA Publishing

Book Cover designed by Linda Arbizu with Claude

1st edition 2024

Dedication

I dedicate this book to my five extraordinary children, Joshua, Benjamin, Miriam, Hannah, and Eve, who gave me the biggest reason to continue living. I love them so much! In addition, I dedicate this book to my mother, Marion, and sister, Ann, who gave me hope and metaphorically talked me off the edge of the cliff, saving my life multiple times. Also, to anyone contemplating suicide, my heart is with you. Please live on and grace us with your unique spark! You are the reason I wrote this book.

Contents

Chapter 1
Facts

United States Statistics

- Suicide is a leading cause of death and affects people of all ages. Suicide is a serious public health problem and has far-reaching impact. Resources are available to prevent suicide. Hope is possible. **https://www.cdc.gov/suicide/facts/index.html**

- Suicides outnumbered homicides in the US from 2011–2020. https://www.samhsa.gov/mental-health/suicidal-behavior/about

- The US suicide rate has climbed 36% over the past two decades (2000-2021) and increased an additional 2% from 2021-2022= 38% increase since 2000. https://usafacts.org/articles/how-is-the-suicide-rate-changing-in-the-us/

- 12.3 million Americans seriously thought about suicide in 2021 — with men, LGBTQ youth, American Indian and Alaska Native people, and veterans at higher risk. https://usafacts.org/articles/how-is-the-suicide-rate-changing-in-the-us/

- NIMH highlighted the pandemic's toll on the young as suicide increased among pre-teens and young adults. The researchers identified 5,568 youth who died by suicide during the first 10 months of the pandemic, which was higher than the expected number of deaths had the pandemic not occurred. https://www.nimh.nih.gov/news/science-updates/2023/youth-suicide-rates-increased-during-the-covid-19-pandemic

- Over 49,000 people in the US died by suicide in 2023. 1 death every 11 minutes. https://www.cdc.gov/suicide/facts/data.html

- In 2023, in the US, many adults thought about suicide or attempted suicide. 12.8 million seriously thought about suicide. 3.7 million made a plan for suicide. 1.5 million attempted suicide. https://www.cdc.gov/suicide/facts/data.html

- Among older men, the suicide rate generally increased with age, with men 85 and older having the highest of any age group (55.7 suicide deaths for every 100,000 people). The report also found that firearm-related suicide was much more common in older men. (Same source as next fact)

- Suicide deaths happen throughout the year, but contrary to what many people think, suicides do not peak during the holidays but are actually more common during summer and fall. https://www.aarp.org/health/healthy-living/suicides-rising-among-older-men/

- Suicide was the second-leading cause of death in 2021 for people ages 10-14 and 25-34 and the third- and fifth-leading cause of death for people ages 15-24 and 35-44, respectively. Between 2020 and 2021, suicide rates increased in every age cohort except for the 45-54 group. https://usafacts.org/articles/how-is-the-suicide-rate-changing-in-the-us/

- In 2021, white people have the most suicide deaths, but American Indians and Alaska Native people have the highest suicide rates for age-adjusted rates per 100,000 people by race/ethnicity. https://usafacts.org/articles/how-is-the-suicide-rate-changing-in-the-us/

- American Indian, Alaska Natives, and Indigenous Peoples communities are placed at a higher risk due to historical trauma, and compounding discrimination and oppression, in conjunction with a lack of investment into supportive resources. https://988lifeline.org/help-yourself/americanindian-a

laskanatives-indigenouspeoples/

- Preventing and Responding to Suicide Clusters in American Indian and Alaska Native Communities Report examines suicide clusters within American Indian and Alaska Native communities. It discusses effective prevention strategies, and offers resources to communities to decrease the prevalence of these clusters. https://library.samhsa.gov/product/preventing-and-responding-suicide-clusters-american-indian-and-alaska-native-communities

- In 2023, the suicide rate among males was nearly 4 times higher (22.8 per 100,000) than among females (5.9 per 100,000). https://www.nimh.nih.gov/health/statistics/suicide

- In 2023, suicide methods: 27,300 used a firearm; 12,023 used suffocation, 5,944 used poisoning; 4,089 used other methods. https://www.nimh.nih.gov/health/statistics/suicide

Global Statistics

- More than 720 000 people die due to suicide every year.

- Suicide is the third leading cause of death among 15–29-year-olds.

- Seventy-three per cent of global suicides occur in low- and middle-income countries.

- The reasons for suicide are multi-faceted, influenced by social, cultural, biological, psychological, and environmental factors present across the life-course.

- For every suicide there are many more people who attempt suicide. A prior suicide attempt is an important risk factor for suicide in the general population.

- The link between suicide and mental disorders (in particular, depression and alcohol use disorders) and a previous suicide attempt is well established in high-income countries. However, many suicides happen impulsively in moments of crisis with a breakdown in the ability to deal with life stresses, such as financial problems, relationship disputes, or chronic pain and illness.

- In addition, experiencing conflict, disaster, violence, abuse or loss and a sense of isolation are strongly associated with suicidal behavior. Suicide rates are also high among vulnerable groups who experience discrimination, such as refugees and migrants; indigenous peoples; lesbian, gay, bisexual, transgender, intersex (LGBTI) persons; and prisoners.

- Stigma, particularly surrounding mental disorders and suicide, means many people thinking of taking their own life or who have attempted suicide are not seeking help and are therefore not getting the help they need... only a few countries have included suicide prevention among their health priorities and only 38 countries report having a national suicide prevention strategy. An individual suffering from depression is twenty times more likely to die by suicide than someone without the disorder. All the global facts above are from https://www.who.int/news-room/fact-sheets/detail/suicide

- Suicide remains illegal in over 20 countries, while people who engage in suicidal behavior may be punished in some countries that follow Sharia law, involving legal penalties that range from a minor fine or short prison sentence to life imprisonment. https://www.iasp.info/wspd/references/

If you are struggling with mental health issues, https://www.samhsa.gov/mental-health call the SAMHSA National Helpline for free, confidential, 24/7, year-round call treatment referrals 1-800-662-HELP (4357)

If you are thinking about harming yourself or attempting suicide, tell someone who can help immediately. Call 911 for life-threatening physical emergencies; Call or text 988 the Suicide and Crisis Lifeline for behavioral health crises that are not immediately life-threatening.

Chapter 2
Why Suicide?

Permanent Solution to a Temporary Problem

"Linda," declared Terry, "Suicide is a permanent solution to a temporary problem." "Yeah," I countered, "But when someone is considering ending it all, they don't believe it is a temporary problem. They cannot see an answer to their dilemma. I know from experience.

Two-Years-Old

The first time I tried to kill myself, I was two years old. I kept running under the streetcars in Essen, Germany, and the nice policeman would bring me back time after time to our apartment, asking whether or not my mom wanted 'this one' because there were five other children in the household. Most German families had one or two kids, not six, which was how many we had at the time."

More Attempts Later

"You can't be sure you were trying to kill yourself. Maybe you were exploring or trying to run away," Terry rebutted. "That's possible," I said, "but that's when the satanic ritual victimization began, and the sexual abuse became more frequent. In addition, I attempted to kill myself a few more times throughout my life, so I know I was trying to get away from pain."

The first secret for you is to understand WHY someone might want to commit suicide. Then, you know where to begin when helping prevent suicide and emotionally supporting a person considering ending their life, even if that someone is you.

Suicide Risk

Suicidal thoughts are a harrowing aspect of human experience, often stemming from a complex interplay of various components, which the Center for Disease Control has categorized for us here as four factors increasing suicide risk:

1. Individual risk factors include previous suicide attempts, a history of mental illness, childhood trauma, chronic pain, job or financial loss, legal problems, violence, and substance use.

2. Relationship risk factors come from hurtful interactions with others, such as bullying and violence, social isolation, loss of relationships, and family suicides.

3. Community risk factors are structural and social issues, such as lack of access to healthcare, community suicide cluster, violence, trauma, and discrimination.

4. Societal risk factors involve cultural and environmental factors, such as a stigma against mental illness, easy access to lethal means for those at risk, and unsafe depictions of suicide in media. https://www.cdc.gov/suicide/factors/index.html

Maslow's Hierarchy of Needs

Understanding a person's "Why?" is essential to provide practical support and intervention. What are people's basic needs? Often, people FEAR losing what they have or FEAR not getting what they want. Maslow's Hierarchy says we have physiological needs (air, water, food, shelter, sleep, clothing, sex), safety (protection from elements, security, order, law, stability, freedom from fear, employment, resources, health, property), love and belonging (friendship, intimacy, family, trust, acceptance, and connection), esteem (dignity, achievement, respect, mastery, independence, status, recognition, prestige), and self-actualization (realizing personal potential, self-fulfillment, growth and peak experiences).

Expanded Models

Expanded models introduce cognitive needs (knowledge and understanding, curiosity, exploration, need for meaning and predictability), aesthetic needs (appreciation and satisfaction through the pursuit of beauty, balance, order, and form through art, music, nature etc.), and transcendence needs (beyond self-actualization, motivated by values transcending the self, service to others, connection with a higher reality, purpose, or the Universe). Information from the Simple Psychology.org website. https://www.simplypsychology.org/maslow.html#The-expanded-hierarchy-of-needs

Survival

The human brain's design is for survival. If we fear not meeting our needs, our body ramps up the adrenaline and cortisol for fight, flight, freeze, or fawn. It is your privilege to alter your thinking patterns and feelings set for mere survival, transform your state, and take action to make yourself happy. It is your job to look for assistance because we need professionals, families (whatever that version looks like), and communities. We are social creatures. It's not only okay to ask for help; it is your responsibility.

Mental Health Disorders

Suicidal ideation and mental health disorders such as depression, bipolar disorder, and schizophrenia are often linked together. These conditions distort thinking, making problems seem insurmountable and solutions nonexistent.

- For instance, depression can engulf you in a shroud of hopelessness and worthlessness, severely impairing your ability to see beyond the current pain.
- Bipolar disorder, with its extreme mood swings, can lead to impulsive decisions, including suicide during depressive phases.

- Schizophrenia can potentially create a distorted reality and drive you towards suicide in an attempt to escape your perceived threats or voices.

Trauma

Trauma, both physical and emotional, is another critical contributor. Those who have experienced traumatic events such as abuse, violence, sexual assault, or severe loss may view suicide as an escape from the relentless flashbacks and emotional turmoil that plague them. Post-Traumatic Stress Disorder (PTSD), a common aftermath of trauma, can significantly increase suicidal tendencies.

Life Stressors

Life stressors: relationship issues like being bullied or losing a loved one, financial problems like losing a job or getting into overwhelming debt, chronic illness with constant physical pain, or lacking access to healthcare when you need it can also lead to suicidal thoughts. These situations can make you feel trapped and desperate, especially when you lack the coping mechanisms or support systems to navigate through them.

Internal Turmoil, Isolation, and Hopelessness

Intense emotional turmoil often marks the internal experience of those contemplating suicide. This inner battle is frequently invisible to outsiders, making it difficult for them to understand the depth of the struggle. This conflict results in profound isolation, an extreme feeling that you are being a burden to others and accompanies a deep-seated sense of hopelessness about the future. In addition, the injury experienced isn't just emotional; it often manifests physically, contributing to a constant state of distress.

Validate Their Pain

Recognizing and validating their pain is crucial. This validation offers a sense of being seen and understood, which can be a critical step in healing. It's important to acknowledge that their feelings, however overwhelming, are valid and understandable given their circumstances. They don't need a lecture. They need understanding and compassion. As they verbalize what's inside, they may see their own solutions. This approach paves the way for effective intervention, establishing trust and opening communication lines.

Compassion

Even if it appears that someone is only seeking attention, show empathy by directing them to professional resources that will help them, at least 988. However, maintain your boundaries to avoid getting pulled into a situation beyond your ability. On the other hand, if a perpetrator tries to manipulate you, show yourself compassion by cutting off all communication with them. Don't get involved with trying to save your offender, or you will find yourself entangled in a web of violence.

Victim-Persecutor-Rescuer Drama Triangle

Compassion for yourself means maintaining healthy boundaries. Doing that can avoid some relationship risk factors for suicide. You may feel stuck in the victim-persecutor-rescuer drama triangle, but hope exists. You can create healthy relationships by challenging and changing your victim into an empowered individual, the persecutor into a self-accountable person, and the rescuer into an authentic supporter. A good depiction of this triangle is from the lindagraham-mft.net website. https://lindagraham-mft.net/triangle-victim-rescuer-persecutor-get/

Mental Health Professionals

Professional support is mandatory in addressing these underlying causes. If you have thoughts of harming yourself, get professional help. Mental health professionals can help you unpack the complexity of emotions and thoughts that contribute to suicidal ideation. Therapy, medication, and support groups are among the tools that can provide relief and coping strategies.

Destigmatize Mental Health Issues

Moreover, societal efforts to destigmatize mental health issues play a vital role. Education and open conversation about mental health can create an environment where people feel safe to seek help, including workplaces, schools, and families, where stressors often first become evident. It's a collective responsibility to provide a safety net for those teetering on the edge, reminding them there is always a path forward, no matter how dark it seems.

Compassion and Comprehensive Approach

Suicidal thoughts are a multifaceted issue requiring a compassionate, comprehensive approach. By understanding the risk factors and underlying causes, which needs they fear being unmet, recognizing the internal struggle and isolation, and validating pain compassionately without dropping boundaries, we can offer hope and support to those who feel despairing and forsaken.

Why and How Else You Can Meet Your Needs

If you are contemplating suicide yourself, you must figure out why you feel that way, what you fear losing, or what you fear not getting. It is your job to ask for help. You have the power to change your thinking patterns and feelings so you can take action to transform your life. But you must ask. It's okay to get help. I have been to so many kinds of therapy, and I am still alive because I had others help me figure out my "why" and how to address it.

Remember, the first secret for you is to understand WHY someone might want to commit suicide. Then, you know where to begin when helping prevent suicide and emotionally supporting a person considering ending their life, even if that someone is you.

End Suffering

"Terry, I just wanted to end my suffering," I replied. "That's why I wanted to die. I couldn't take any more physical, emotional, and spiritual pain. Even after my near-death experience from the car accident, and I knew better, I still tried one more time because of the illusion that it would cease the torment and agony, and the emotions were too overpowering." Terry hugged me and said, "Well, I am grateful you got some therapy and are here now for me to love!"

Chapter 3

What is Suicide's Lie?

Activated Charcoal

"Linda, wake up and drink this," the emergency room technician said. "Where am I? What is this stuff that you want me to drink?" I mumbled in a groggy state. "It's activated charcoal," Anna answered. "We just pumped your stomach, and this will bind with the residual toxins so you can defecate them out." "Why did you do that, damn it?" I asked belligerently.

Anna

"How old are you?" Anna asked. "I'm twenty," I replied. "You are so young. Why would you do this to yourself?" I recited the inner dialogue, "My boyfriend is still married to someone else, sleeps with anyone he wants, tells me about it, and still I love him. It hurts so much. I need him to love me, but he doesn't, and no one wants me. They only want sex. I want the pain to stop."

Many Reasons

The last chapter discussed the rationale why a person might consider killing themselves and the risk factors involved. If you have known someone or are someone who has thought about killing yourself, you know there are many reasons why a person might consider it. The bottom line is that suicide promises to stop the misery.

The Deception of Relief

I want to shred suicide's lie that it will end whatever torment a person at risk is experiencing, giving the illusion of relief because it doesn't deliver. It's a dirty deception! The person who dies may not feel anything more physically in this life, but they will have to karmically balance the suffering they throw onto those who loved them when they have their life review. In addition, I am becoming aware of the universe within me and my responsibility to those entities. This life is not the end!

The second secret for you is to realize that suicide will not provide the relief sought because we carry the same vibrational energy and consciousness into the afterlife. Because of my 1997 near-death experience, I can tell you that whatever vibration you have at death is the one you will carry into the afterlife. If you think death is the termination of your intellectual unit, you are mistaken. Now, while you are alive in this body, is the time to change your vibration to be more harmonious with the purpose for which consciousness/your higher power/the quantum field created you. I know it may seem impossible to escape the despair, but with help, you can rise above it—with hope. You deserve to live— and to live happily!

Other's NDEs

Near-death experiences (NDEs) provide compelling anecdotal evidence for the continuity of consciousness. Frequently, people who experience NDEs report remarkably similar experiences regardless of their cultural or religious backgrounds. These experiences typically include a feeling of being detached from the body, encountering a brilliant light, a sense of overwhelming peace, and sometimes interactions with perceived spiritual entities or deceased loved ones.

Continuity of Consciousness

One of the most intriguing aspects of NDEs is the reported clarity and heightened awareness during these experiences, even in cases where individuals were clinically dead or in situations where expected brain function is severely impaired or non-functional. Such accounts challenge the conventional understanding that consciousness is solely a product of brain activity. Medical professionals and researchers have been documenting and studying NDEs for decades. While some say this is not definitive "proof," these experiences propose that consciousness extends beyond the physical brain and death.

Psychology

In psychological terms, consciousness associates itself with the mind's workings – thoughts, memories, emotions, and perceptions. The exploration of altered states of consciousness, such as those experienced in deep meditation, psychedelic experiences, and, indeed, near-death experiences, has expanded the understanding of consciousness. Transpersonal psychology, in particular, delves into aspects of consciousness that transcend the individual, suggesting a more expansive, interconnected nature of awareness that persists beyond physical existence.

Spirituality

Spirituality largely embraces the idea of an enduring consciousness through your non-physical essence, sometimes called the soul or spirit, that animates human beings. Metaphysical authorities view your essence as your eternal aspect, unbound by the constraints of the physical world. Many spiritual traditions emphasize the development of this inner essence because the afterlife's vibrational state reflects the energy cultivated during your life, advocating a direct correlation between your earthly existence and what you experience after you die.

Science

Quantum physics introduces us to the tiniest units that scientists can observe as they interact with the Zero Point field: "The Einstein equation was simply a recipe for the amount of energy necessary to create the appearance of mass. It means that there aren't two fundamental physical entities – something material and another immaterial – but only one: energy. Everything in your world, anything you hold in your hand, no matter how dense, how heavy, how large, on its most fundamental level boils down to a collection of electric charges interacting with a background sea of electromagnetic and other energetic fields - a kind of electromagnetic drag force. As they would write later, mass was not equivalent to energy; mass was energy. (McTaggart, P.33)

Quantum Mechanics

In physics, this concept is evident in the study of quantum mechanics, where we see particles as wave functions, vibrating and fluctuating constantly according to their interplay with "the field." According to Wikipedia.org, quantum mechanics is the study of matter and its interactions with energy on the scale of atomic and subatomic particles. https://en.wikipedia.org/wiki/Introduction_to_quantum_mechanics

Quantum Mind and Consciousness

The "quantum mind" hypothesis proposes that quantum phenomena, like entanglement and superposition, could be integral to the functioning of the brain and consciousness. While still a subject of debate and ongoing research, it introduces the fascinating possibility that consciousness might be a fundamental, quantum-based aspect of the universe, potentially surviving beyond the death of the physical body. I have been there. Consciousness is energy that can neither be created nor destroyed.

Government

The CIA's declassified Analysis and Assessment of the Gateway Process on 9 June 1983, using hypnosis, biofeedback, transcendental meditation, and quantum mechanics to describe the nature and functioning of human consciousness, was a "...training system designed to bring enhanced strength, focus and coherence to the amplitude and brainwave frequency of brainwave output between the right and left hemispheres so as to alter consciousness, moving it outside the physical sphere so as to ultimately escape the even the restrictions of time and space." In other words, they taught people how to expand their consciousness outside their bodies for war purposes. https://www.cia.gov/readingroom/docs/cia-rdp96-00788r001700210016-5.pdf

You Are a Living Energy Field

According to Healthline.com, under the What We Know tab, "You are a living energy field. Your body is composed of energy-producing particles, each... in constant motion. So, like everything and everyone else in the universe, you are vibrating and creating energy... (in) a kind of rhythm. Rhythms happen on a grand scale, like seasonal changes and tidal patterns. They also happen within your body... (like) heartbeats, breathing rates, (and) circadian rhythms." https://www.healthline.com/health/vibrational-energy#what-we-know

What Affects Your Vibrational State?

The interconnectedness of thoughts and words, emotions and moods, and actions or behaviors with your vibrational state is crucial to understanding energy dynamics. Of course, various other factors affect your vibrational state, like physical environment, social relationships, music, visual stimuli you experience, etc., but they are outside of you. Here, we examine what's within.

Thoughts and Words

Thoughts are not just abstract concepts; they are energy forms with a life of their own that influence your vibrational frequency, and when you speak them, they are even more potent. Positive thinking, focusing on gratitude, kindness, and love, raises your vibration, while negative thoughts like catastrophic thinking or verbalizing gossip can lower it. However, positive thinking without action that reinforces your good idea will leave you feeling betrayed and become detrimental, so you have to act on your new goals or beliefs to follow through and build self-trust.

The Vibrations of Emotions

The scientific view coalesces with spiritual perspectives that every emotion has a unique energy frequency that indicates your current vibrational state. On reddit.com, in a discussion on David Hawkins's emotional scale, "At the low end of the spectrum, one can see this energy manifest and express itself as states associated with shame, lust, stress, apathy, etc. You find drive, laughter, joy, serenity, visionaries, trailblazers, reason, love, and the like at the high end of the spectrum. Different energy levels correspond to each of these. ...Hawkins created a map for us... to navigate these states." https://www.reddit.com/r/mentalhealth/comments/wd6snu/the_david_hawkins_scale_navigating_emotional/?rdt=55610

Moods

Moods are merely prolonged habitual emotions. It's valuable to recognize that our emotional state and mood often respond to our thoughts and perceptions, creating a feedback loop with our vibrational energy. There is no doubt that it takes effort to move up the emotional scale from where you are, but how long you decide to remain in a negative emotional state is up to you.

Actions or Behaviors

Actions or behaviors, meanwhile, are the physical manifestations of your thoughts, words, emotions, and moods. They have the potential to significantly impact your vibration, both in the immediate sense and over time. Acts of kindness and compassion are high-vibrational, enhancing not only your energy but also positively affecting those around you. Conversely, actions stemming from negative emotions can contribute to a lower vibrational state.

Interconnected Field of Energy and Universe

Delving deeper into hard science, psychology, and spirituality offers a broader understanding of vibrational energy and consciousness. Modern physics, particularly quantum mechanics, has begun to explore concepts that resonate with psychology's expanded consciousness and spirituality's ancient wisdom. The quantum field theory suggests that everything in the universe is part of a vast, interconnected field of energy, echoing the psychological view of entwined awareness and the spiritual view of an indivisible universe.

Why Subjective Experiences?

From a scientific standpoint, experts often see consciousness as a byproduct of the brain's complex processes. However, the complicated problem of consciousness— the question of how and why we have subjective experiences— remains unresolved. Some scientists and philosophers propose that nonlocal consciousness might be a fundamental aspect of the universe, much like space and time, conveying that it has vibrational qualities.

Consciousness and Vibrational Energy

Near-death experiences offer compelling anecdotal evidence that consciousness and physical existence are not inextricably tied together. Insights from psychology suggest a more expansive understanding of consciousness, while spirituality has long embraced the notion of its continuity through the soul or spirit. Scientifically, consciousness affects and is affected by vibrational energies through quantum mechanics.

Vibrational Energy Shapes Vibrational State

Exploring vibrational energy helps bridge the gap between vibrational states and the continuity of consciousness. Our thoughts and words, emotions and moods, and actions or behaviors are more than just fleeting or subjective experiences; they are dominant tools that shape our vibrational state and, by extension, our conscious reality in this life and beyond.

Again, The second secret for you is to realize that suicide will not provide the relief sought because we carry the same vibrational energy and consciousness into the afterlife. Because of my 1997 near-death experience,

I can tell you that whatever vibration you have at death is the one you will carry into the afterlife.

Now Is the Time

If you think death is the termination of your intellectual unit, you are mistaken. Now, while you are alive in this body, is the time to change your vibration to be more harmonious with the purpose for which consciousness/your higher power created you. I know it may seem impossible to escape the despair, but with help, you can rise above it—with hope. You deserve to live— and to live happily!

Love Yourself

"Look, sweetie," Anna counseled. You may not believe it now, but if you get some therapy, you will most assuredly find someone to love you as soon as you begin to love yourself. And read some books about overcoming co-dependence."

Chapter 4
Warning Signs and Communication

Walt

"What have you been doing today?" asked Walt. I hesitated. "Do you honestly want to know?" I answered with a question. "Well, yeah. That's why I asked," he responded. "The last time I talked to you, you didn't sound like you were doing very well." I answered with a question to deflect his focus, "Well, how are you doing? He replied, "I'm doing alright. I found a few more places to prospect a couple of miles from my place, and I've got a customer wanting to buy the processing machine I designed and built that can use water or air to separate the gold after it crushes the rocks."

Google Search

"That's wonderful!" I said, trying to muster up enough enthusiasm to sound believable. "You still haven't answered my question," he prodded. "What have you been doing?" "Well," I googled whether it was better to shoot yourself in the head or the heart if you want to guarantee that the shot will be fatal. I have seen people who ended up shooting half their face off but didn't die, and I don't want to end up like that."

The third secret for you is recognizing warning signs and using empathic communication. Suicidal ideation involves thinking about, considering, or planning suicide. The transition from ideation to planning or attempting suicide can be swift, making early recognition urgent. Especially if the behavior is new, has increased, or seems related to a painful event, loss, or change, you may want to explore resources quickly or call 988 for immediate help.

Warning Signs

According to the 988lifeline.org website https://988lifeline.org/learn/warning-signs/ The most evident signs are: verbal declarations (talking about: wanting to die, feeling hopeless, feeling trapped, feeling like a burden), actively searching online for ways to kill themselves or buying a gun, shifts in social interactions (withdrawing or isolating), mood changes (anxious, agitated, or reckless) , increased drug or alcohol use, sleeping too little or too much, showing rage or seeking revenge, and extreme mood swings.

- **Verbal Cues**

- Sometimes, individuals may verbally express their thoughts about not wanting to live or feeling hopeless. They may even joke about ways they are going to kill themselves. These expressions should always be taken seriously. They might say:

  I wish I weren't here.
  Everyone would be better off without me.
  I'm just going to kill myself.
  I feel so hopeless about _______.
  I have no reason to live.
  I'm trapped.
  I can't take the pain.
  I am such a burden to ________ (parents, family, partner, friends, etc.)

- **Actively Looking for Ways to Kill Themselves**

They might search online for whether a gunshot to the head or heart is more lethal, or painless, deadly poisons, or how long it takes to die from exhaust asphyxiation, or buy a gun, or get access to other fatal means.

- Social Withdrawal

Withdrawing from friends, family, and social activities is a common sign. Isolating themselves, they make excuses for why they "can't make it" to every social event you invite them to. The person may feel like a burden to others, preferring isolation over social interaction.

- **Changing Mood**

They may exhibit mood swings or lose interest in previously enjoyed activities. They may act uncharacteristically nervous, anxious, or agitated. Paying attention to such changes is vital, especially following significant life events like losing a loved one, a relationship breakup, or major career changes.

- **Risky Behaviors**

There might be an increase in risky behaviors, such as reckless driving: excessive speeding, taking sharp turns, tailgating, and driving while intoxicated. They may be unusually promiscuous or otherwise engage in unsafe sexual practices. They may make unusual choices that might be a cry for help or show a lack of concern for their well-being.

- **Increasing Drug or Alcohol Use**

They may start to need a little "nip" before breakfast or "wake and bake," or disappear for long periods without an explanation or show up wasted, hammered, tanked up, fried, loaded, or toasted for work or other activities that they didn't before because they just needed to "take the edge off" now that something stressful has happened in their lives.

- **Sleeping too little or too much**

Their sleeping patterns might be different, like sleeping excessively, or maybe they have insomnia and cannot sleep at all. They might lose their appetite and find an excuse to leave the table or skip a meal. Or they might have just the opposite problem of overeating compulsively. These can all be indicative of deeper issues. A noticeable decline in personal care or neglect of responsibilities can also be a red flag.

- **Showing Rage or Seeking Revenge**

They may be enraged, throwing things around, slamming doors, yelling and hollering about getting revenge, fighting impulsively, or talking about vengeful acts like vandalism or assault.

Use the 5 Action Steps

Again, from the 988Lifeline.org website, "These evidence-based action steps provide a blueprint for reaching and helping someone in crisis. 1) Ask. 2) Be there. 3) Help keep them safe. 4) Help them connect. 5) Follow up." https://988lifeline.org/help-someone-else/

Empathic Communication Strategies

Do's and Don'ts

Talking with and finding help for someone who may be suicidal can be difficult. Here are some tips that may help:

1. Be direct. Talk openly and matter-of-factly about suicide.

2. Be willing to listen. Allow expressions of feelings. Accept the feelings.

3. Be non-judgmental. Don't debate whether suicide is right or wrong or whether feelings are good or bad. Don't lecture on the value of life.

4. Get involved. Become available. Show interest and support.

5. Don't dare them to do it.

6. Don't act shocked. This will put distance between you.

7. Don't be sworn to secrecy. Seek support.

8. Offer hope that alternatives are available but do not offer glib reassurance.

9. Take action. Remove means, like weapons or pills.

10. Get help from people or agencies specializing in crisis intervention and suicide prevention. https://988lifeline.org/help-someone-else/

Practice Active Listening

Hearing someone talk differs from actively listening to what that person is saying. Active listening requires concentration and understanding. It's more about understanding the person's feelings and perspective than solving their problems. Improving your listening skills is easy with practice and these helpful ideas.

Acknowledge the Speaker

This can be as simple as a nod or an "Uh huh." By acknowledging the speaker, you are letting them know that you are listening to what they have to say and reminding yourself to pay attention to what is being said so you can remember it later.

Respond Verbally

Asking questions or making statements may help clarify what they are saying. It reminds them that you listen attentively, are here to support them, and are genuinely concerned. Be sure to let the speaker finish talking before asking any questions.

Summarize What You Hear

Reflecting on their words is also a positive verbal, active listening technique. Repeating, paraphrasing, or even summarizing what they have said shows you are trying to understand them better. Use phrases like; "what I'm hearing is..." or "sounds like you're saying...." These tactics can also allow them to hear what they are saying, which may help them find positive reinforcement.

Look the Part

Keeping eye contact, maintaining good posture, and staying focused are key components of active listening and interpersonal communication. Being distracted and unfocused gives the speaker the impression that you aren't paying attention.

Let Them Know You Care

When you actively listen to someone, you let them know that you care about what they are saying, indicating that you are concerned for their health and safety. These tips are from the 988lifeline.org page on helping someone else. https://988lifeline.org/help-someone-else/

Non-judgmental Approach

Approach the conversation without judgment. Avoid dismissing their feelings or minimizing their problems. Phrases like "You have so much to live for" might be well-intentioned but can feel dismissive. Focus instead on acknowledging their pain and letting them know you are there to listen.

Open-Ended Questions

Ask open-ended questions encouraging discussion, such as, "How have you been feeling about what's been happening in your life?" or "What can I do to support you right now?"

Validate Their Feelings

Validation doesn't mean agreeing with their thoughts of suicide but acknowledging that their feelings are authentic and valid. Saying, "It sounds like you're in a lot of pain," or "I can see how that situation would be tough for you," can be very comforting.

Offering Support and Resources

Let them know that help is available, and that seeking professional support is a sign of strength, not weakness. Offer to assist them in finding a therapist, contacting a crisis line, or even going with them to a doctor's appointment.

Safety Planning

If someone is in immediate danger, do not leave them alone. Remove any potential means of self-harm if possible and seek immediate professional help. In some cases, this may mean calling emergency services (911) or (988) if they are willing to talk to a suicide prevention professional.

Empathy and awareness are indispensable in dealing with individuals showing signs of suicidal ideation. Recognizing the warning signs and engaging in empathetic communication can make all the difference. It's important to remember that while we can offer support and listen, professional help is necessary at some point, and encouraging or facilitating access to such assistance can be life-saving.

Sensitivity

Remember, conversations about mental health should be approached with sensitivity and care. It's not just about preventing a crisis but also about fostering an environment where seeking help and expressing feelings is normalized and encouraged. The third secret for you is recognizing warning signs and using empathic communication.

No Gun Right Now

"Okay, Linda," said Walt, "You don't have a gun out right now, do you?" "No," I responded. "I am sure it's nothing. I have dealt with these feelings all my life, like a bad habit. It's just sometimes it gets too intense." Walt ended, "Good, I'm glad you don't have a gun out. I'll be over in half an hour to take you to lunch so we can talk a little more. Okay? Maybe I can bring you to my place afterward to see my new pug puppies."

Chapter 5
Contacting 988

KaDe

"Who are you talking to?" I inquired. "None of your business! Get out of here!" yelled my big sister KaDe as she stretched the phone cord until she could sit on the stairs with the door closed. Before cell phones, we had only one phone attached to a wall in the house, so we could always hear each other's conversations. She was fifteen, and I knew she was unhappy, but it sounded like she was on the suicide crisis line again. I was worried about her but didn't know how to help. "Would you like a glass of water?" I asked. "Okay," she answered, "I am thirsty."

The fourth secret for you is to know what to expect when you contact 988 and how to help on social media. On July 16, 2022, the 988 Lifeline transitioned away from the National Suicide Prevention Line, reached through a 10-digit number, to the three-digit 988 Lifeline. It is funded by the Substance Abuse and Mental Health Services Administration (SAMHSA) and administered by Vibrant Emotional Health (Vibrant). Professionals will still service the old number for those who have yet to learn about 988.

What to Expect

When people call, text, or chat with the 988 Lifeline, they are connected to trained crisis counselors who are part of the existing 988 Lifeline network of over 200 local crisis centers operating since 2005. These crisis counselors are trained to provide free and confidential emotional support and crisis counseling to people in suicidal crisis or emotional distress and to connect them to resources. These services are available 24 hours a day, seven days a week, across the United States.

Automated Greeting

After dialing 988, an automated greeting will address you and ask you to respond after it plays. Then the system sorts you to the correct crisis counselor: "You have reached the 988 Suicide & Crisis Lifeline, also serving the Veteran Crisis Line. Para Español oprima el número dos. (If the caller presses "2," they are routed to the Spanish sub-network.) If you are in emotional distress or suicidal crisis or are concerned about someone who might be, we are here to help."

Current Military or Veteran

If you are a US military veteran or current service member or are calling about one, please press 1 now. (If the caller presses "1," they are routed to the Veteran Crisis Line). Otherwise, please hold while we route your call to the nearest crisis center in our network.

Waiting Music Plays

Music plays while the phone system routes the call to the closest crisis center in the Lifeline network based on area code. Each crisis center picks its coverage area (which can be defined by zip code, area code, county, or even state) and its hours of operation.

Trained Counselor Answers

A trained crisis counselor at a local center will answer the phone. (If the local center cannot answer, the call is routed to the national backup network.) This person will listen to the caller, work to understand what the caller is experiencing, provide support, collaborate with the caller on ways to feel better and connect with any needed help or resources. https://988lifeline.org/get-help/what-to-expect/

Chat

When someone uses the Lifeline chat via https://988lifeline.org/chat/, they first complete a short survey letting the crisis counselor know a little about their current situation. Then, they see a wait-time message while connecting to a crisis counselor.

Text

When someone texts 988, they will complete a short survey letting the crisis counselor know a little about their current situation. They will then be connected with a trained crisis counselor, who will interact with them to understand what the texter is experiencing, provide support, and connect them with any needed help or resources.

Support on Social Media

For over ten years, the 988 Suicide & Crisis Lifeline has worked with social media platforms and digital communities to establish recommended best practices in suicide prevention for social and digital media. All information below is from https://988lifeline.org/help-someone-else/safety-and-support-on-social-media/

Safety Processes on Social Media:

If you are worried about someone on social media, you can contact safety teams, who will reach out to connect the user with the help they need. *Note: Tumblr no longer directly responds to reports of suicide or self-harm.

Facebook- Report suicidal content here: https://www.facebook.com/help/contact/305410456169423From reporting to supporting video here: https://vimeo.com/160565004

Twitter- Twitter will send the user a direct message with the Lifeline number. Click here to report messages about suicide or self-harm to Twitter. https://help.twitter.com/en/forms/safety-and-sensitive-content/self-harm

Instagram- To report posts about suicide or self-harm on Instagram: Tap "..." below the post, Tap Report Inappropriate, Select This Photo Puts People At Risk > Self-Harm.

Snapchat- To report a safety concern, press and hold onto that Snapchatter's name and tap the gear button. Then, tap 'Report,' reach out to Snapchat, and follow the prompts. https://help.snapchat.com/hc/en-us/requests/new?start=5153567363039232

YouTube- To report suicide or self-harm, click "More." Highlight and click "Report" in the drop-down menu. Click "Harmful dangerous acts," then "Suicide or self-injury." YouTube will review the video and may send a message to the uploader with the Lifeline number.

Discord- Use the drop-down in Discord's report form to report self-harm and select 'Trust & Safety.' Under 'Report Type,' select 'Self-harm.' Discord requests that you verify the report's authenticity by providing a link to the message where the user expresses such harm. You can find the steps below. https://support.discord.com/hc/en-us/requests/new?ticket_form_id=360000029731How to contact Discord Safety for Parents and Guardians article here: https://support.discord.com/hc/en-us/articles/360000291932

TikTok- To report for self-harm on TikTok, tap the arrow at the bottom right-hand corner of the video. Tap the report icon, select "Self-injury," and follow the prompts. Here is an article explaining what to do if you see a user who needs support: https://newsroom.tiktok.com/en-us/what-to-do-if-you-see-a-user-who-needs-support/

Reddit- If you're worried about someone, you can let Reddit know by reporting the specific post or comment that worried you and selecting "Someone is considering suicide or serious self-harm." After you let them know, they'll reach out (confidentially) to put the user in touch with Crisis Text Line's trained Crisis Counselors. Article What do I do if someone talks about seriously hurting themselves or is considering suicide?

https://support.reddithelp.com/hc/en-us/articles/360043513931-What-do-I-do-if-someone-talks-about-seriously-hurting-themselves-or-is-considering-suicide-

Pinterest- If you come across a pin or comment that is concerning to you, learn how to report Pinterest content here: https://help.pinterest.com/en/article/report-something-on-pinterest

Directions for Twitch, X, and Bluesky can also be accessed at https://988lifeline.org/help-someone-else/support-on-social-media/

Identify Suicidal Crisis

One of the first hurdles to cross in establishing a process for suicidal community members is one of identification. How do you know if someone may be in a suicidal crisis? Examples of a community post from someone who may be at risk are like this:

- "Hi, I really need some help. Can someone please contact me?"
- "My daughter has fibromyalgia, and the treatment alone costs too much for us to keep up with everything else. It's become a full-time job to take care of her, and I don't know how to keep going like this. I feel hopeless with all this and don't know how to keep going."
- "My 15-year-old son has been texting one of his friends, and he has been having what appears to be thoughts of suicide. What should I do?"
- "I've been really depressed lately, and I don't know how to deal with this. I have been thinking about suicide lately; my grandfather committed suicide ten years ago. I'm so scared about all of this."

Identified But Not Imminent Risk

Suppose you have identified an individual who is at risk of suicide or in a suicidal crisis but doesn't seem to be at imminent risk. In that case, research suggests that the community moderator reach out to that individual directly through a set of explicit processes established by and best suited to the needs of your platform or community.

Not Mental Healthcare Professionals

While we encourage active moderation and response online, we do not encourage community managers to take on the role of mental health care professionals. All engagement with an at-risk individual should be designed to provide appropriate support while connecting that individual to mental health or crisis resources like the Lifeline, your local crisis center, or other local mental health providers.

Call 911 For Urgent Risk

If you believe that a person may genuinely be at urgent risk of suicide (like if they have already taken pills or have a gun in their hand), call 911 or other local emergency services for immediate assistance. Local emergency services are the fastest way to help someone right now. Other resources or protocols may be inappropriate and should not be applied during this situation.

All information on this page is excerpted from https://988lifeline.org/help-someone-else/safety-and-support-on-social-media/

The fourth secret for you is to know what to expect when you contact 988 and how to help on social media.

Below is a list of global crisis lines for countries around the world. I don't know how they work, but it's a place to begin if you aren't in the United States.

https://en.wikipedia.org/wiki/List_of_suicide_crisis_lines

https://faq.whatsapp.com/1417269125743673/?locale=en_US

Conversation With KaDe Continued

"Here is your water, KaDe," I said as I offered her the plastic cup. "Thanks, Linda," she verbalized to me. "Hey, does it really help you feel better when you talk to these people? I inquired. "Yeah," she asserted, "Sometimes it's easier to talk to strangers than family or friends because they don't judge you so much when you talk about this stuff. You know what I mean?" I didn't understand exactly what she meant because she was using some words I didn't know on the phone, but she was my big sister, and I figured she must know everything, so I nodded yes.

Chapter 6
Navigating Crisis Moments

JoAnne

"JoAnne, what's going on? Why aren't you going to class?" I questioned as I saw her walk behind the high school building. Her big blue eyes were bloodshot and red, and tears streamed down her fifteen-year-old cheeks. She hadn't been to drama class for a few days, and I knew she was ditching again, but I was really concerned about her this time. I knew she had a rough family life. "I don't want to talk about it?" she retorted. "Come on, you can tell me," I prodded.

Mom Didn't Believe Me

"Well, you know, my stepdad," she blurted out, "I told you about him before. He keeps coming into my room at night and getting in bed with me. He hurts me. I tried to tell my mom, but she didn't believe me, and she slapped me across the face. What am I supposed to do? I can't get any sleep to think up a way to stop him. My brain hurts, and I am so scared. Sometimes, I think it would be better for my mom if I were dead. Maybe I should just kill myself."

The fifth secret for you is creating and implementing a safety plan for crisis moments. Navigating a suicidal crisis requires both immediate coping strategies and a long-term plan.

<u>Strategies for Coping During Acute Suicidal Crises</u>

1. **Recognizing the Crisis Brewing**

The initial step in navigating through a suicidal crisis involves recognizing and acknowledging you are in a critical state without minimalizing or rationalizing. A surge of intense emotions characterizes this phase, which may include profound despair, feelings of worthlessness, and recurrent thoughts of self-harm or suicide. Understanding and accepting that these feelings and thoughts indicate you are in a crisis is vital.

2. **Finding Immediate Distractions**

Distractions can serve as a potent, immediate strategy to cope with the overwhelming emotions and thoughts experienced during a suicidal crisis. The objective of using distractions is to temporarily divert attention away from your distressing thoughts and provide a mental break. Activities that demand cognitive engagement or physical exertion can offer a different focus.

- Calming or uplifting music- Listening to calming or uplifting music can be soothing and help shift your mood. Try listening to classical music like Mozart or Yoga Station instrumental music. You might like how calm it makes you feel.

- Engaging in physical movement- Walking, running, bicycling, hiking, dancing, yoga, qigong, Pilates, or exercising in whatever way you want— releases endorphins, dopamine, serotonin and other neurotransmitters, which are natural mood lifters. Find a way to exert yourself physically.

- Doing mental or creative activities- Putting together puzzles or filling in Sudoku boxes can distract you. You can also start doing creative activities like drawing, painting, making a collage with old magazine pictures (we did that in the old days), writing, playing an instrument, or singing, which can also provide a constructive outlet for your emotions and thoughts.

3. **Using Grounding Techniques**

Grounding techniques are practical tools that help reconnect you with the present moment, thus helping reduce the intensity of overwhelming emotions. These techniques focus on utilizing the senses to anchor your awareness in the 'here and now' instead of being lost in the trauma of the past or fear of the future.

- Deep breathing exercises can induce a state of calm and help in managing panic and anxiety. Box breathing: exhale for a count of four, hold lungs empty for a count of four, inhale for a count of four, hold the air in lungs for a count of four, and begin the pattern anew. Here are some other breathing exercises to try as well. Alternate nostril breathing, belly or diaphragmatic breathing, 4-7-8 breath, lion's breath, mindfulness breathing, pursed lip breathing, and resonance breathing are explained on this website: https://www.verywellmind.com/abdominal-breathing-2584115

- Mindfulness practices like body scan meditation or guided imagery encourage focusing on the current experience without judgment, which can relieve distressing thoughts. Make sure not to listen to these while driving or operating machinery. Listen while sitting or lying in a comfortable position and a safe space.

    - Body scan meditations help you reground or center yourself by bringing your full attention to physical sensations and experiences. Here is an example of a ten-minute body scan meditation on this website. https://www.youtube.com/watch?v=uqtIqCKjkuc

    - Guided imagery or visualization meditations use your imagination in a relaxing place like a beach, meadow, mountaintop, park, desert, or fishing, and all five senses to relax your body. Here is an example of guided imagery, twenty-two-minute Eye Movement Desensitization, and Reprocessing safe place binaural beat meditation to listen to with headphones on. https://www.youtube.com/watch?v=IQI82AvvWNI

- Sensory-focused activities, such as holding a piece of ice in your hand; chewing gum or crunchy foods; running your hands through sand, grass, or water; playing with playdough; hugging yourself; massaging your head, arms, legs, and feet, gently brushing your skin with a soft brush on your arms, legs, or head; or rocking back and forth on a swing or soft couch. These can redirect your mind's attention from suicidal thoughts to your physical sensations. Here is an eleven-minute EMDR visual of a blue butterfly moving across the screen without music activity. https://www.youtube.com/watch?v=DheesiCVbK8

4. **Reaching Out to Someone**

In moments of acute crisis, especially when your emotions are overwhelming, reaching out for support is foremost. Contacting a trusted friend, family member, or a mental health professional can prove life-saving. Call 988 if you don't want to "bother" anyone else. That is what these trained crisis counselors do. Their professional help can supply immediate intervention and guide you to manage your crisis further. Sometimes, talking about what you are experiencing can alleviate the situation's intensity. You are worth it!

IASP

Here is another resource from The International Association for Suicide Prevention for two other hotlines on what to do when you are in a suicidal crisis or if you are supporting someone in a suicidal crisis. https://www.iasp.info/suicidalthoughts/

Guidelines to Create a Personalized Safety Plan

Using distractions, grounding techniques, or sensory-focused activities may help feelings subside, but if they don't, get help. Once you recognize warning signs, implement your safety plan. If you still need to create one, take the time to do it when you are stable. If you are already in a crisis, you may need to move to a safer environment, use other coping strategies, or call a designated support person. It is important to remember that these painfully intense feelings are temporary and manageable with proper support and strategy.

1. Custom-made and Practical

A safety plan is a personalized, practical plan that includes ways to stay safe and steps to take during a suicidal crisis. Design it when you are calm and can think clearly, ideally with the assistance of a mental health professional. Please put it in your phone or write it down to see the steps precisely outlined when you are in a crisis and might have trouble thinking.

2. Identify Your Triggers and Warning Signs

Part of the safety plan should involve identifying your triggers and warning signs that a crisis might develop, such as specific thoughts, feelings, situations you find yourself in, or behaviors you do. Observe your warning signs and write them in your plan. They can vary but often include increased hopelessness, intense emotional pain, withdrawing from others, or engaging in risky behavior.

- Are you frequently crying for seemingly no reason? Do you eat compulsively or stop eating altogether? Is it difficult to get out of bed, or do you have trouble sleeping? Do you drive too fast, drink too much, or break things? Write them down because these are your personal triggers. Knowing your warning signs can help you take action before a crisis escalates.

3. Steps to Take During a Crisis

The plan should list actions and the steps you commit to doing when a crisis hits. Include distraction techniques that personally help you redirect your thinking, like holding a piece of ice or massaging your head, grounding exercises like breathing exercises or mindfulness meditations with their accompanying website links that work best for you, or discover music that makes you feel serene and put it on your phone as well, and finally, prepare a list of whom you feel comfortable contacting for support. Explore your options when calm and clear-headed before you find yourself in crisis mode. Always remember, if nothing else is working, call 988.

4. Emergency Contacts List

A crucial element of the safety plan is an emergency contacts list. The contacts list should include the numbers of close friends or family members, your therapist or other mental health professionals, and crisis hotlines. Have them readily available on your phone or written down on a card in your wallet if you don't have your phone for some reason.

5. Accessible and Reviewed Regularly

Ensure the safety plan and contacts list are easily accessible. Again, please keep them on your phone or a small card in your wallet, and you can review them regularly to keep them up-to-date. If you try something that doesn't work, delete it from your plan and add something else. Keep many options handy so you have all your bases covered. If someone changes their number or only wants you to text, write it down in your plan so you don't have to try to remember it in a crisis.

The fifth secret for you is creating and implementing a safety plan for crisis moments. Navigating a suicidal crisis requires both immediate coping strategies and a long-term plan. By understanding and recognizing your unique warning signs, having a clear and accessible safety plan, and knowing whom to contact in an emergency, you empower yourself to be prepared to handle a crisis.

Open to Hope

The key is to remember that even in despair, you can take steps to ensure your safety and seek help. Prematurely ending your life is avoidable, and having a strategy to manage your crisis moments is a crucial part of that prevention. Your personal safety plan is a valuable tool to enact when you feel out of control. Through preparedness, support, and the willingness to reach out, navigating through crisis moments can lead to recovery and hope.

School Counselor

"JoAnne, let's talk to the school counselor. She might be able to make him stop," I offered. "But they would call the cops, and my mom would never forgive me for ratting out my stepdad," claimed JoAnne. "Well, you can't keep living like this. Your mom should be protecting you from him. That's why they have laws and police and stuff. Let's go talk to the counselor before you end up doing something you really didn't mean to do."

Chapter 7
Prevention

Indigenous People

"So all the substance use disorder support groups (wow, that's a mouthful) you facilitate for the Tohono O'odham people are online?" I queried. "Yup," Ann answered, "We have many different kinds of people joining the group, but most are court-ordered. Our group is pretty structured to meet the state requirements, so I present a topic like 'What activities can you do instead of using your substance,' and their assignment is to make a list before we meet again to discuss it as a group. Sometimes, the things people share are pretty intense.

Intense Experiences

One teenage kid lives with his uncle because his parents are in jail for dealing drugs. Last week, his uncle overdosed and died. He had one cousin shoot himself last year, and another hang himself three months ago." "Wow," I remarked, "How come?" "Well," said Ann, "There are many reasons, but these are broken people. There is a lot of death, drugs, alcoholism, intergenerational trauma, poverty, and limited access to healthcare—not to mention the restricted availability of healthy food or clean water. Something like 90% of people are diabetic, and depression and substance use disorders are pretty common too."

Prevention

For those considering suicide, the primary drive is to escape unbearable pain, whether emotional, psychological, or physical. Averting suicide involves identifying and employing long-term strategies that can alleviate this pain in healthier, more sustainable ways. We discussed handling crises in the last chapter, but now, let's examine other longer-term prevention methods.

The sixth secret for you is to locate a longer-term therapist, use online resources, watch videos, and find the right support group to help you avoid crises. At one time, society stigmatized therapy to be only for sickly, incompetent, or "crazy people." However, now we know that therapy is a good idea for everybody because we live in a confusing time and society, and those at risk for suicide will benefit immensely from entering therapy.

Close the Gratitude Loop

There is no shame in getting help! Receiving is the highest form of giving because it closes the gratitude loop. Someone has to accept and receive for another to give, so you allow someone to feel the joy of giving when you receive. In addition, using resources like therapy or support groups is not a weakness but a strength, demonstrating your resourcefulness and self-love. Good for you!

Mental Health Resources and Therapeutic Approaches

1) Locate a Professional Therapist

Therapy can be a safe space to explore feelings, identify underlying issues, and develop coping strategies. "Speaking to someone... can help you feel better and improve mental health," says the 988lifeline.org help yourself section. https://988lifeline.org/help-yourself/

- Your Medical Insurance Carrier—If you have insurance, the first place to start is by calling or online chatting with your carrier. Be bold and ask. They can provide a list of therapists covered under your policy, which will cost less than other resources. Look at the card for the phone number or website.
- The healthline.com website, under therapy for every budget, has

recommendations and reviews for diverse approaches. It gives a quick look at the best affordable therapy resources. https://www.healthline.com/health/therapy-for-every-budget#A-quick-look-at-the-best-affordable-therapy-resourcesThe review links on the site show how much the services cost and why they picked it.

- **Most flexible:** Talkspace https://talkspace.pxf.io/c/411371/1425671/14729?rvo_aff=1&rvo_brandid=Talkspace&rvo_prodid=9055d50d-83d9-47b1-a1bb-4d54138c8644&rvo_subid=9055d50d-83d9-47b1-a1bb-4d54138c8644&rvo_subid2=%2Fhealth%2Ftherapy-for-every-budget&subid1=null&subid2=/health/therapy-for-every-budget&subid3=19d7a16f-e1cf-4198-a92a-fe8678c7ed01
- **Best for those with insurance:** Grow Therapy https://growtherapy.com/?rvo_aff=1&rvo_brandid=Grow+Therapy&rvo_prodid=044f5999-20fa-4af9-9c5b-e9a0c2e3a9fa&rvo_subid=044f5999-20fa-4af9-9c5b-e9a0c2e3a9fa&rvo_subid2=%2Fhealth%2Ftherapy-for-every-budget&correlationId=f658dc25-2d14-4b9d-8936-a262f7571feb
- **Best for those without insurance:** Open Path Psychotherapy Collective https://openpathcollective.org/?rvo_aff=1&rvo_brandid=Open+Path+Psychotherapy+Collective&rvo_prodid=b5f09fd6-b562-46b7-afbd-571b61a96c46&rvo_subid=b5f09fd6-b562-46b7-afbd-571b61a96c46&rvo_subid2=%2Fhealth%2Ftherapy-for-every-budget&correlationId=36b551e9-4930-4afb-99bb-300f3c76c60f

- **Best for financial aid:** BetterHelp https://impact.betterhelp.com/c/411371/3769750/39552?rvo_aff=1&rvo_brandid=BetterHelp&rvo_prodid=e673de28-62ed-4e85-983b-16b82dc8461b&rvo_subid=e673de28-62ed-4e85-983b-16b82dc8461b&rvo_subid2=%2Fhealth%2Ftherapy-for-every-budget&subid1=null&subid2=/health/therapy-for-every-budget&subid3=795ada3d-32a4-4e92-bba3-de60522974a6

- **Best for couples:** OurRitual https://impact.ourritual.com/LKzY4j?rvo_aff=1&rvo_brandid=Our+Ritual&rvo_prodid=3516bae3-8fb3-44c1-b8e2-e3bf95525eb8&rvo_subid=3516bae3-8fb3-44c1-b8e2-e3bf95525eb8&rvo_subid2=%2Fhealth%2Ftherapy-for-every-budget&subid1=null&subid2=/health/therapy-for-every-budget&subid3=d52fffe7-4544-4e26-8c53-245065ca6b93

- **Best subscription variety:** Calmerry Online Therapy https://calmerry.sjv.io/c/411371/3062827/36808?rvo_aff=1&rvo_brandid=Calmerry&rvo_prodid=0627b954-73e4-47f5-93ac-5b8a28586d83&rvo_subid=0627b954-73e4-47f5-93ac-5b8a28586d83&rvo_subid2=%2Fhealth%2Ftherapy-for-every-budget&subid1=null&subid2=/health/therapy-for-every-budget&subid3=c9dcb404-f336-4c0f-b704-da00c0e28bb9

- **Best for online and in-person sessions:** Octave Therapy https://www.findoctave.com/individual-therapy?rvo_aff=1&rvo_brandid=Octave+Therapy&rvo_prodid=238d8c20-2dc2-49dc-851e-f426bbeae5f4&rvo_subid=238d8c20-2dc2-49dc-851e-f426bbeae5f4&rvo_subid2=%2Fhealth%2Ftherapy-for-every-budget&correlationId=ce5d7f28-95e4-4e59-8bca-e43771c56a81

- The resources below are listed directly from the 988lifeline.org website under help yourself, Find a Therapist/Support Group. https://988lifeline.org/help-yourself/

- **SAMHSA Mental Health Services Locator. https://findtreatment.samhsa.gov/**
- **Psychology Today Therapist and Support Group Finder. https://therapists.psychologytoday.com/rms/**
- **American Foundation for Suicide Prevention Suicide Bereavement Support Group Finder. https://afsp.org/find-support/ive-lost-someone/find-a-support-group/**
- **Therapist Finder through Online Therapy. https://www.onlinetherapy.com/**
- **Inclusive Therapist Finder. https://www.inclusivetherapists.com/**

They cater to the "needs of those with marginalized identities: Black, Indigenous, and People of Color (BIPOC) and LGBTQIA2S+ intersections (QTBIPOC). Their website says, "Our mission prioritizes the voices and expressions of Neurodivergent and Disabled Communities of Color."

There are resources for all people- Neurodivergent, Youth, Veterans, Attempt Survivors, Black Mental Health, Disaster Survivors, Loss Survivors, Deaf or Hard of Hearing, Maternal Mental Health, Native American/Indigenous/Alaska Natives, and LGBTQI+ people can find help at the inclusive therapists' website.

- Online therapy- You can find specialists of many kinds: Cognitive Behavioral, Anger Management, Anxiety, Christian, Divorce, Eating Disorder, Long-distance Relationships, African American Therapists, Online Addiction, Online Anxiety, Online Career Counseling, Online Life Coaching, Online Marriage Counseling, Online Premarital Relationships, Psychiatrists (medication), Online Sex Therapy, Online Self-esteem Therapy, Suicide Prevention Therapy, Trauma and Post-traumatic Stress Disorder Therapists and others https://www.onlinetherapy.com/ There is even an option for free sessions, but there are restrictions. https://ww

w.onlinetherapy.com/free/

Types of Beneficial Therapy

Known types of therapy beneficial for suicidal ideation include cognitive-behavioral therapy (CBT), dialectical behavior therapy (DBT), psychodynamic therapy (PDT), and internal family systems therapy (IFST). They help develop coping mechanisms, reframe negative thinking, and process traumatic experiences so you can manage suicidal thoughts and the underlying issues that fuel them.

2) Medication

In some cases, medication may be necessary to treat underlying mental health conditions like depression or anxiety. Antidepressants, mood stabilizers, anti-anxiety medications, or other psychotropic pharmaceuticals prescribed and monitored by a psychiatrist can be part of an effective treatment plan. I was on antidepressants for thirty-seven years. Then, I took a break for four years and started back on them last year. There are some psychedelics also gaining approval for use for depression and PTSD. Personally, I have done Spravato treatments (a derivative of Ketamine) for a year now and have had excellent results. Ask your psychiatrist if some of these new treatments might be good for you.

3) Online Resources and Support Groups

We already discussed 988, available 24/7, but mental health websites or online support groups can also offer information and community support. Like in-person support groups, online groups can provide camaraderie and peer support when needed.

- **Online Depression Support Groups**

According to Healthline's Best Online Support Groups for Depression https://www.healthline.com/health/mental-health/online-depression-support-groups#A-quick-look-at-the-best-online-support-groups-for-depression "A 2015 study found that 15 participants in an online depression support group felt participation helped decrease their symptoms and self-stigma during a 10-week period. The study found that participants valued communication with others in a judgment-free zone and, in some cases, felt more comfortable talking about their depression with 'strangers' in the group than with their family and friends."

- **Best for frequent engagement:** Anxiety and Depression Association of America. https://healthunlocked.com/anxiety-depression-support

- **Best for support on the go:** Bezzy Depression. https://www.bezzydepression.com/?rvo_aff=1&rvo_brandid=Bezzy&rvo_prodid=1d7d47df-9d3d-4436-92a6-258cf8ec4209&rvo_subid=1d7d47df-9d3d-4436-92a6-258cf8ec4209&rvo_subid2=%2Fhealth%2Fmental-health%2Fonline-depression-support-groups&correlationId=026d51b5-c55a-440b-8250-9bc899eb363f

- **Best for 24/7 support:** 7 Cups. http://www.7cups.com/?rvo_aff=1&rvo_brandid=7+Cups&rvo_prodid=743572b6-ce8f-40ce-81c2-96292de099f9&rvo_subid=743572b6-ce8f-40ce-81c2-96292de099f9&rvo_subid2=%2Fhealth%2Fmental-health%2Fonline-depression-support-groups&correlationId=e4aa0b98-3fb1-4318-aad4-0c3d9b0a3d68

- **Best for virtual meetups in your neighborhood:** NAMI Connection. https://www.nami.org/Support-Education/Support-Groups/NAMI-Connection?rvo_aff=1&rvo_brandid=National+Alliance+on+Mental+Health+%28NAMI%29&rvo_prodid=6d4cab79-fc3d-4d61-b701-ebc79b2b6aef&rvo_subid=6d4cab79-fc3d-4d61-b701-ebc79b2b6aef&rvo_subid2=%2Fhealth%2Fmental-health%2Fonline-depression-support-groups&correlationId=46c81f33-4c59-47e7-8487-0825276c303e

- **Best for specialized support groups:** The Depression and Bipolar Support Alliance.

https://www.dbsalliance.org/support/chapters-and-support-groups/online-support-groups/?rvo_aff=1&rvo_brandid=Depression+and+Bipolar+Support+Alliance&rvo_prodid=63cd28d8-10cd-43e5-b402-8bcd7283f742&rvo_subid=63cd28d8-10cd-43e5-b402-8bcd7283f742&rvo_subid2=%2Fhealth%2Fmental-health%2Fonline-depression-support-groups&correlationId=3bff1a35-d149-4d38-8141-aa030b3932a4

- **Best for co-occurring mental health concerns:** Inspire by Mental Health America. https://www.inspire.com/groups/mental-health-america/topic/depression/?origin=tfr&rvo_aff=1&rvo_brandid=Mental+Health+America&rvo_prodid=27378d95-c808-45fd-bbd3-9001ad28a3bd&rvo_subid=27378d95-c808-45fd-bbd3-9001ad28a3bd&rvo_subid2=%2Fhealth%2Fmental-health%2Fonline-depression-support-groups&correlationId=65be4804-b479-4337-97d9-af9f7d710d4d
- **Best for postpartum depression:** Postpartum Support International. https://www.postpartum.net/?rvo_aff=1&rvo_brandid=Postpartum+Support+International&rvo_prodid=e50d2dce-a7d0-4ac9-968c-2a982372e9da&rvo_subid=e50d2dce-a7d0-4ac9-968c-2a982372e9da&rvo_subid2=%2Fhealth%2Fmental-health%2Fonline-depression-support-groups&correlationId=fdaf2d8d-e96e-4b27-8060-e25d77bece3c
- **In the Rooms Global Recovery Community and Meetings.** https://www.intherooms.com/home/category/community-and-meetings/

4) YouTube videos on Suicide Prevention Playlist. https://www.youtube.com/playlist?list=PLlvnz6vjrZYdxPz2AgcnKoTwgt3eXYwu1

5) Self-Care During the Holidays List. https://988lifeline.org/self-care-during-the-holidays/

Take a walk outside.
Write a love letter to yourself.
Write about something you are grateful for in your life (it can be a person, place, or thing).
Create a happy playlist and a coping playlist.
Treat yourself to a favorite snack.
Watch your favorite movie.
Forgive someone.
Forgive yourself.
Say, thank you to someone who has helped you recently.
Create a DIY self-care kit of things that make you feel better.
Take your medication on time.
Take a new fitness class at the gym (yoga, Zumba, etc.).
Plan a lunch date with someone you haven't seen in a while.
Pamper yourself with an at-home spa day.
Take a day off from social media and the Internet.
Reach out to your support system.
Cuddle with your pets or a friend's pet.
Take the time to stop, stand and stretch for 2 minutes.
Wake up a little earlier and enjoy your morning cup of tea or coffee before the morning rush.
Take a hot shower or bath.
Take yourself out to dinner.
Volunteer.
Start that one project you've been contemplating for a while.
Sit with your emotions, and allow yourself to feel and accept them. It's okay to laugh, cry, and feel whatever you're feeling with no apologies!
Cook a favorite meal from scratch.
Take a 5-minute break in your day.
Compliment someone (and yourself, too!)
Permit yourself to say no.
De-clutter your mind: write down five things that bother you, then throw them away.
Donate three pieces of clothing that you no longer wear.

Take the time to find five beautiful things during your daily routine.
Take a mental health day from school, work, etc.
Take a nap.
Reach out to the Lifeline.

6) Video Success Stories of Hope and Recovery. https://988lifeline.org/stories/

There are inspiring success stories of others who have been in similar situations and faced a suicidal dilemma, but they overcame their thoughts of self-harm and now flourish just like you can. I enjoyed these stories and felt very uplifted.

Be Open and Willing to Try Different Strategies

What works for one person may not work for another. Therefore, it's wise to keep an open mind and be willing to try different strategies. Finding the right combination of treatments you can afford, and practices you will keep up with, is profoundly personal and requires patience and perseverance. Your happiness is worth it! Keep going!

Strength

It's important to remember that seeking professional help is a sign of strength, not weakness. Locating a longer-term therapist, proper medication, using online resources like forums, watching videos that may provide guidance, and finding a support group are all methods that can be the winning preventative solution.

The sixth secret for you is to locate a longer-term therapist, use online resources, watch videos, and find the right support group to help you avoid crises. Your journey toward healing may have ups and downs, but with the right strategies and resources, a path to a healthier, more peaceful life is achievable. Remember, you are not alone; with time and support, healing and hope are within reach—with hope.

Conversation With Ann Continued

"You would think the Tohono O'odham Nation would implement some kind of treatment plans for the youth if there is so much suicide." I declared. "Well, that's why the young man I was talking about is in my substance use disorder group, but there is widespread denial of the problem because people think that 'talking about suicide will make it happen' or that the person 'just wants attention' or 'it will pass,' or 'there's nothing anyone can do when someone makes that choice,' or 'it won't happen in strong families.' It's sad, and I am doing my best for the people in my group, but I really worry about this kid."

Chapter 8
Thriving After Surviving Trauma

Andrea

My therapist, Andrea, begins, "Okay, Linda, let's focus on the first time you were afraid for your siblings since you said that was particularly distressing. Sit comfortably and close your eyes. Can you see the situation? How old were you?" "Probably about two," I muttered. "Where are you?" "We are in a basement below the basement where they kept coal in our apartment building in Germany," I responded.

Eye Movement Desensitization and Reprocessing (EMDR)

"Pay attention to your body's sensations, emotions, and how these change as we view the event. I will tap on your forearms with this amount of pressure alternating from your right to left arms. Is that pressure okay?" asked Andrea. I nodded. "You can stop me anytime you need to, alright? You are safe here with me in the therapy room." I nodded again.

Continued Tapping

"How are you feeling as you see this situation?" she requested. "I am sad." Andrea taps alternating forearms and asks, "Now, what are you feeling?" "Powerless," I answered. Andrea keeps tapping as I start to cry...

The seventh secret for you is prioritizing caring for your body and mind so that you can thrive after trauma. In chapter two, we learned that some individual risk factors include childhood trauma, chronic pain, and violence, which can contribute to current trauma. Post-traumatic growth (PTG) is a term that refers to the positive psychological change you can experience from adversity and other challenges. You rise to a higher level of functioning, which includes a greater appreciation for life, new possibilities in life, enhanced personal strength, and spiritual development.

Caring For Your Body and Mind in a New Loving Way

The foundation for growing from trauma comes from caring for your body and mind in a new, loving way and reframing your trauma. These acts of self-love can improve your physical health, mood, and overall mental health.

1. The Psychosomatic Relationship

The connection between body and mind is profound. Mental health issues can manifest physically, and physical health problems can affect mental well-being. Understanding this bidirectional relationship is crucial in holistically treating physical and psychological health. Regular health check-ups, adequate sleep, and managing physical ailments are necessary because poor physical health can exacerbate mental health issues, potentially triggering or worsening depressive symptoms and suicidal thoughts. Holistic approaches like massage and acupuncture can complement traditional treatments to promote well-being.

2. Nutrition and Mental Health

Understanding the deep connection between the physical and the mental is critical in addressing the root causes of depression and suicidal ideation. Nutrition plays a vital role in mental well-being. Experts say diets rich in vegetables, fruits, whole grains, lean protein, and omega-3 fatty acids are linked to better emotional health. Conversely, diets high in processed foods, sugar, and unhealthy fats can negatively impact mood and energy.

3. Exercise as a Natural Antidepressant

Exercise is a potent tool in combating depression and suicidal ideation. It releases endorphins, natural mood lifters, and reduces stress hormones. Regular physical activity, whether brisk walking, yoga, qigong or more intense exercise, can significantly improve mood and mental health. I watched a video introducing me to Egoscue pain-free exercises that you can access for free on YouTube- Realign By Randee. Here is the link for her Necks Cervical spine video: https://www.youtube.com/watch?v=0OpKqPgtXlg

- More Free Resources: I also like Marisa with Yoqi on YouTube for getting chi flowing correctly through your body. https://www.youtube.com/watch?v=nmmNWj9YtAw Mathew Sanford with Mind Body Solutions.org also has free adaptive yoga classes for those who are disabled. https://www.mindbodysolutions.org/video-hub/

- Moving your body awakens your life force energy and reduces chronic stress, which can lead to both physical and psychological health problems, including increased risk for depression and suicidal thoughts. Managing stress through physical activity and healthy lifestyle choices is indispensable.

4. Self-Compassion Creates a Positive Self-relationship

Caring for your mind begins a positive self-relationship. Positive affirmations in the mirror (Louise Hay's "Mirror Work") and being compassionate with yourself generate confidence and develop your positive self-relationship. Treating yourself with the same kindness, concern, and support you would show a good friend as you acknowledge your suffering without judgment lets you trust yourself more.

- Think kind thoughts about yourself- When experiencing suicidal thoughts, harsh self-criticism and negative self-talk destroy your relationship with yourself. Self-compassion encourages a gentler, more understanding approach to struggles and failures. Also, set a little goal and accomplish it. When I was stuck in the hospital bed on my back for two months, I used the foam triangle thing between my legs to rock back and forth until I could get up on my side to put a bedpan under me. I only had my left arm working, so it was tricky, but I celebrated not having to wait for a nurse's aide to relieve myself.

- Chanting new beliefs- I am also learning more about chanting new beliefs with a strong emotional expression, feeling it deeply within your body from Tony Robbins. He says walking or exercising while chanting new beliefs like "I am powerful" or "I am enough" will help cement them into your self-identity. The idea is that you have to get your body and your emotions engaged to change your beliefs. https://www.youtube.com/watch?v=m2ix1iAbbfc

5. Tools For Positivity

We previously discussed meditation, which can give inner peace, increase your vibrational state, and help you become more aware of yourself without condemnation. You can also write yourself a letter from the perspective of a compassionate friend so you can verbalize your feelings and support yourself emotionally, or keep a gratitude journal. Reflecting daily on what you are grateful for will shift your focus from negative to positive aspects of life.

- Go outdoors- In addition, the natural beauty and serenity of the outdoors enhance your vibrational state, so take time in nature to bring serenity, reduce stress, and improve your mood. Relax, pursue a hobby or creative activity, socialize with loved ones, or volunteer to feel fulfilled. These things can provide hope and positivity.

6. Better Relationships and Mental Health

Self-compassion leads to better relationships with others because as you treat yourself with kindness, you desire to extend that to others (with healthy boundaries in place) and attract people who will do likewise with you. Studies also show that self-compassion reduces depression, anxiety, and stress. You improve mental health by compassionately addressing negative thoughts and emotions and teaching yourself to be patient with setbacks, build emotional resilience, a positive outlook, healthier relationships, and reduce symptoms of mental health disorders.

7. Reappraise Traumatic Events

You can show self-compassion through cognitive reappraisal, changing your thoughts about a past traumatic event. Instead of viewing it solely as a source of pain, you can see it as a catalyst for growth, learning, and resilience. You may find strength by assigning new meaning to your trauma through therapy or journaling. You might help others who have gone through similar experiences or channel the experience into creative or professional endeavors. Trauma survivors reframe their story from one of victimhood to one of survival and growth. I love the saying that life happens FOR you, not TO you!

8. Discover Purpose and Meaning in Life

After reappraising your traumatic events, discovering your purpose and creating meaning in life might happen automatically. If they don't, you may realize that you don't have just one purpose. Maybe surviving and thriving are some of your goals. You don't have to lock yourself into just one direction or implication. Life perpetually changes, and you can redefine meaning and purpose in each new moment.

- Inner Work- You may need to do some inner work, but you can do it because you are worth it! The human spirit thrives on having a reason to live, a goal to strive for, and a belief in the value of one's existence. You'll have a more positive outlook on life because you feel a sense of direction, self-worth, and resilience, shifting focus from pain and suffering to goals and aspirations. In finding purpose, you not only enrich your life but often touch the lives of others, creating ripples of positive change and hope.

- Self-reflection and introspection—This can help identify personal values, passions, and strengths. Questions like "What brings me joy?" and "What am I good at?" can guide this exploration.

- Experimenting with new activities—Exploring different interests out of your comfort zone effectively uncovers hidden passions and potential purposes, such as volunteering, taking up a new hobby, or traveling.

- Insightful feedback—Ask friends, family, or mentors to offer perspectives on your strengths and talents and how these might be applied in meaningful ways to help clarify a purpose.

The Artist Who Turned Pain into Passion

Jane, a young woman struggling with depression and suicidal thoughts from being sexually abused as a child, discovered painting as a form of therapy. Through her art, she found a way to express her emotions and realized her purpose in advocating for mental health through her artwork. Her exhibitions began to showcase her journey and inspired others to find healing in creativity.

Transforming Pain into Purpose

Mike's story is another example of post-trauma thriving. Post-recovery from his suicidal phase, he turned to marathon running, channeling his pain into physical endurance challenges. His journey inspired many and raised awareness about mental health and the importance of physical activity in recovery.

The Student Who Overcame Adversity

Lily, a college student, faced severe anxiety and suicidal ideation after being raped on campus. She started therapy, got on medication, began to exercise, and ate a more healthy diet, so she began to heal. She found purpose in helping others facing similar challenges and started a campus support group that created a community that fostered healing and hope for herself and her peers.

Opportunities For Growth

The concept of post-traumatic growth offers a hopeful perspective for those recovering from suicidal thoughts and trauma. It suggests that while trauma can leave deep scars, it also presents opportunities for remarkable personal growth, resilience, and a renewed sense of purpose. By understanding and nurturing the intricate relationship between the body and mind, you can get healthcare, eat well, exercise, develop self-compassion and positivity, build better relationships, reappraise traumatic events, and find purpose and meaning to combat depression and overcome suicidal thoughts.

Thrive Through Body and Mind Self-Care

Beyond merely surviving trauma, there lies the possibility of thriving - creating a more vibrant, meaningful life filled with a deeper understanding of yourself and the world. The seventh secret for you is prioritizing caring for your body and mind so that you can thrive after trauma, having the courage, support, and willingness to see beyond the pain and embrace the transformative power of your experiences.

Continuation of EMDR Session With Andrea

"Okay, Linda. Did you feel a shift or a release in your emotional state as you view the event now?" "Yeah, I feel a little calmer," I answered. "Let's stop and drink water and go to the bathroom, and then we'll come back and find a new, positive belief or emotion about the event to cement into your mind, okay? I will do the same tapping as I did before. I'll see you in a few minutes."

Chapter 9
Your Relationship With Yourself is Foremost

Group Therapy

"The topic for our group today," announced Maddie, the group facilitator, "is some simple things you can do to take care of yourself emotionally so you don't get stuck in the downward spiral of negative thinking. Mary, let's start with you." "I can go kill that bitch that stole my husband!" exploded Mary. "I understand you are outraged, Mary, and I am sure you have valid reasons to be angry, but today, we want you to focus on yourself. What can you do with Mary, for Mary, that would show her that you love her and want to take care of her?" questioned Maddie.

Simple Things

"Well, I like to listen to music and dance in my room. Is that what you mean?" replied Mary. "Yes," Maddie said. "That's what I mean. How about you, Alex?" "I like running or drawing," answered Alex. "Good. How about you, Mike?" continued Maddie. "I like meditating. And I want to take a shower today," said Mike. "I like to feel the sun on my face and collect seashells on the beach," April volunteered.

The eighth secret for you is to create a healthy relationship with yourself to reduce your suicide risk. A relationship is the connection, association, or involvement between two or more entities. The fundamental relationship to nurture is one with your different inner entities. What? I am only one entity, you say? Anyone who has had suicidal ideation can tell you that conflicting conversations are going on inside their mind.

Fractured to Protect You

These automatic negative dialogues stuck in your brain were imprinted into you before you were seven by the dysfunctional attachment styles with your earliest caregivers. It wasn't your fault, but it is your job to heal. Initially, your whole, perfect self splintered into parts to perform roles designed to protect you.

Creating a Healthy Relationship With Yourself

The recommendations from the last chapter were about nurturing the whole self with practical tools so you can become physically and mentally healthy. In contrast, this chapter examines those fragmented pieces of you and why they initially split so you can better understand yourself.

Exercise Self-Compassion

Once you understand those pieces and why they split, you will have a solid framework to exercise self-compassion and restore your psyche to health. Once you are more healthy, you can also create vibrant interpersonal relationships with other healthy people, thus reducing your suicidal risks from toxic relationships. But, to begin with, you need to understand yourself.

Internal Family Systems Model

The Internal Family Systems model says different parts of your psyche need to be "unburdened" so you can enjoy compassion, creativity, curiosity, confidence, courage, calm, connectedness, clarity, presence, persistence, perspective, playfulness, and patience qualities of the perfect "Self" before the fragmenting.

***Disclaimer-** If you are mentally ill, delusional, paranoid, or schizophrenic and may not be grounded in reality, this model may not work for you because you may misuse the idea of "parts." You will need a mental health professional to guide you in finding a therapeutic modality that will work better for you.

Three Personality Types of Parts to Unburden

In IFS, you can distinguish the parts of a person that need to be unburdened by three personality groups:

1. Exiles— Exiles are young, vulnerable parts that carry "burdens," kept in isolation by managers or firefighters to protect other parts of the self from experiencing difficult emotions.
2. Managers— Managers are parts that use various proactive ways to protect the individual from being overwhelmed by difficult emotions carried by exiles. Their job is to control the person's psyche and stabilize the system.
3. Firefighters— Firefighters are a group of reactive parts that activate impulsively when the exiles' difficult emotions come to the surface to control them (they extinguish emotional fires).

Exiles

Our parents, the nanny, the babysitter, or whoever took care of you when you were a child "...hurt these young parts of your personality in some way and then (you) got 'stuck' in the past in some 'time-warp...' These (parts) still hold memories of distressing events and carry various emotional burdens... Past trauma, guilt, shameful memories, and 'bad' thoughts are all exiles..."

Denied and Rejected

Our upbringing made us deny our weaknesses and suppress unpleasant feelings. That is why we are vulnerable to trauma... When some parts of us suffer, we refuse them, and thus, they are not only in pain because of the trauma but also left feeling rejected and abandoned by us. That's how they become exiles...

Burdens

The most frequent burdens of the exiled parts are fear (I am not safe), guilt (This is my fault), anger, shame (There is something wrong with me), responsibility, a sense of worthlessness, hopelessness, loneliness, emptiness, grief, and disappointment... Once relieved of the burdens carried by the exiled parts, we can open up to all sorts of experiences and attitudes typical for children, for instance, natural spontaneity, joy, creativity, etc.

Managers

Exiles will do anything to get noticed. Therefore, they will constantly bring back memories and emotions to remind us they are there. They will keep doing this until we give them attention and look after them... Managers run our day-to-day lives by locking up the exiles to maintain the system balance. Managers use phobias, obsessions, compulsions, passivity, emotional indifference, panic attacks, depression, hyperactivity, people-pleasing, overthinking, self-criticism, and nightmares to keep the unwanted exile from surfacing.

Manager Types:

The Controller is the part who wants to have control over everything because it thinks that any unwelcome or unforeseen event will trigger your emotions related to some trauma.

The Perfectionist believes as long as it's perfect, it won't get rejected, and consequently, it will not evoke in you the problematic feeling of being left alone.

The Passive pessimist part avoids interpersonal contact through withdrawal and passivity so as not to get close to other people because closeness can release strong, suppressed emotions.

The Baby-sitter cares about everyone around you, except yourself, and uses this strategy to escape your emotions.

Managers Are "Driven Into" These Roles

These roles the manager takes... are not its essence but rather an extreme role that it was "driven into,"... and a critic can become a motivator if we communicate with it and make it see the damage it is causing with its criticism... We set the exiles free from their emotional burdens during therapy... and managers no longer need to protect us from the emotions that previously threatened us, as they are now healed.

Fire-fighters

In therapy, the firefighter may evoke specific psychophysical reactions in the body, such as drowsiness, dizziness, and distraction, anything that will allow the person to escape from facing what (they are terrified of feeling)...

Must Numb Pain

There are situations when managers can no longer keep exiles away. In such moments, we are overwhelmed by feelings, and such emotional fire needs to be quickly extinguished... They want to numb and ease the intense emotions of the exiles or distract us from them... To minimize pain, Firefighters may fight, flee or freeze no matter the cost.

Self-Harm

They may use extreme strategies like cutting, binging, and purging. They may even want to end life to stop suffering. These parts respond to triggers associated with past trauma (exiled parts) to stop the resulting emotional pain. Examples of firefighter parts include alcohol and drug use, self-harming behaviors, or suicidality.

Addictions

Firefighters have the same goal as managers but assume different roles and strategies. Managers are... "proactive protectors" (they prevent emotions from getting stirred up), whereas firefighters are "reactive protectors" (they activate when the damage is done)... The most common strategies of firefighters are addictive behaviors involving food, sweets, smoking, alcohol, drugs, pornography, gambling, shopping, work, and use of social media. All IFS information I used is from the Michael Past erski.com website. https://pasterski.com/2019/11/types-of-parts-in-ifs/

Parent's Attachment Pattern

Before you were seven, your relationship with your earliest caregivers imprinted an attachment pattern that affects all future relationships, including the one with yourself. "Parents play many different roles in their children's lives, including teacher, playmate, disciplinarian, caregiver and attachment figure. Of all these roles, their role as an attachment figure is one of the most important in predicting the child's later social and emotional outcome," says the NIH National Library of Medicine website. https://www.ncbi.nlm.nih.gov/pmc/articles/PMC2724160/

A Secure Attachment Style

From the Help.org website, we get an idea about what a secure attachment style creates in a child. https://www.helpguide.org/articles/relationships-communication/attachment-and-adult-relationships.htm#:~:text=Disorganized%20attachment-,Secure%20attachment%20style:%20what%20it%20looks%20like,thrive%20in%20close,%20meaningful%20relationships."A secure parent-child attachment relationship tends to establish an empathic child who feels safe, stable, able to set appropriate boundaries, and is more satisfied in their close relationships. While they don't fear being alone, they usually thrive in close, meaningful relationships."

Why Did Your Perfect "Self" Splinter?

Unfortunately, not all parents and early caregivers were emotionally well themselves, so they forged an unhealthy relationship style with their children, which affected the children for the rest of their lives. These are called attachment injuries. You may recognize your parents in one of these descriptions and realize why your infant self coped in the way it did. The NIH National Library of Medicine website shows us four attachment disorders. https://www.ncbi.nlm.nih.gov/pmc/articles/PMC2724160/#:~:text=Of%20the%20four%20patterns%20of,2,18%E2%80%9324

The Four Attachment Disorders

1. Insecure—Loving foundation, but they seek proximity to and maintain contact with the caregiver until they feel safe because the caregiver was inconsistent.

2. Avoidant—An insecure foundation from an insensitive parent who rejects, ignores, ridicules or is easily annoyed. The child develops a strategy for dealing with distress that is also 'organized' in that they avoid their caregiver when distressed, minimize displays of negative emotion in the presence of the caregiver, and avoid the caregiver in times of need.

3. Resistant—This is also an insecure foundation from an insensitive parent who was inconsistent. Infants whose caregivers respond in erratic, unpredictable and 'involving' ways, such as expecting the infant to worry about the caregiver's own needs or amplifying the infant's distress and being overwhelmed, also using an 'organized' strategy for dealing with distress; they display extreme negative emotion to draw the attention of their inconsistently responsive caregiver.

    - Resistant But Organized—The strategy is said to be 'organized' because the child 'knows' exactly what to do with an inconsistently responsive caregiver, i.e., exaggerate displays of distress and use angry, resistant responses, 'hoping' that the inconsistently responsive caregiver cannot possibly miss the marked distress response. However, this resistant strategy is also 'insecure' because it is associated with an increased risk of developing social and emotional maladjustment.

4. Disorganized—These are atypical, insecure, disorganized parental styles. -Approximately 15% of infants in low psychosocial risk and as many as 82% of those in high-risk situations do not use any of the three organized strategies for dealing with stress and negative emotion. These children have disorganized attachments...
    - Atypical Caregivers—"Atypical caregiver behaviors, referred to as 'frightening, frightened, dissociated, sexualized or otherwise atypical,' are aberrant behaviors displayed by caregivers during interactions with their children that are not limited to when the child is distressed. There is evidence to suggest that caregivers who display atypical behaviors often have a history of unresolved mourning or unresolved emotional, physical, or sexual trauma or are otherwise traumatized (e.g., post-traumatic stress disorder or the traumatized victim of domestic violence)."

Resilience Through Self-Compassion

Hopefully, becoming aware of the different parts of yourself and realizing the attachment injuries imprinted from your earliest caregivers before you were seven is why your perfect self splintered will open your heart to the self-compassion you deserve. Resilience through self-compassion is needed to heal your fundamental relationship with yourself from these early wounds.

Strengthen the Skill of Resilience

Positivity, flexibility, and the ability to manage emotions to adapt to adversity effectively give resilience the capacity to endure, learn from, grow, and acknowledge the difficulty of a situation while maintaining hope and working toward recovery. Strengthening this skill allows you to steer through emotional turbulence without being overwhelmed, reducing the likelihood of a crisis escalating to suicidal thoughts. The eighth secret for you is to create a healthy relationship with yourself to reduce your suicide risk.

Back to Group Therapy Ending

Maddie finished, "I think we have covered a few simple things you can do to take care of yourself emotionally today: music, dancing, running, drawing, meditating, showering, feeling the sun on your face, and collecting seashells on the beach. Great job! Tomorrow, we are going to list which of these things, or maybe some new things you can do when you start feeling like you want to harm yourself. See you tomorrow."

Chapter 10

Recovery Dharma For Addictions

AA Meeting

"My name is Bob," stated Bob, "and I am a recovering alcoholic." "Hi, Bob," said the group. "Yeah, I resonate with this first step, admitting we are powerless over alcohol and that our lives have become unmanageable. My wife just took our kids and left me six months ago. I told her so many times I didn't have a problem. I knew I could quit whenever I wanted to. I mean, I didn't even start drinking much until I lost my job. Then I realized it was a problem because I struck my six-year-old son, and I knocked him out. He hasn't spoken to me for six months."

Twelve Steps and Twelve Traditions

Here are the links to the Twelve Steps and Twelve Traditions from the Alcoholics Anonymous website, designed to help you overcome addiction. https://www.aa.org/the-twelve-stepshttps://www.aa.org/the-twelve-traditions

Al-Anon Meeting

Pauline began, "I didn't even realize I had a problem until I learned about codependence and being an enabler. He was the one drinking and drugging. I just kept it hidden because I was so ashamed. I told the kids, the neighbors, and his employer that Joe was sick. I made so many excuses for him. When he blackened my eye, I said I bumped into the door knob while doing laundry. I Googled patching the walls where he put holes, and I told my mom everything was fine, even though I was thinking about killing myself..."

Al-Anon Twelve Steps

Here is the link to the Al-Anon.org website for the Twelve Steps. https://al-anon.org/for-members/the-legacies/the-twelve-steps/

You can find the **Emotions Anonymous Twelve Steps Groups** recovery program for people experiencing anxiety, grief, depression, anger, low self-esteem, and other emotional difficulties on the recovery.org support groups emotions anonymous website. https://emotionsanonymous.org/

The ninth secret for you is to incorporate the Recovery Dharma, Four Noble Truths, and Eightfold Path into your addiction treatment to lessen your suicide risk. If you don't have any addictions at all, this chapter is not for you. However, in my own life, I have found that even suicidal ideation itself was a form of addiction as one of my firefighter parts tried to exile whatever painful emotion was trying to surface: fear (I am not safe), guilt (This is my fault), anger (This is unfair), shame (There is something wrong with me). Other miserable states include feeling like I'm not fulfilling responsibilities, a sense of worthlessness, hopelessness, loneliness, emptiness, grief, and disappointment.

Suffering is the Story Created From Emotional Pain

According to the livingsystems.ca website, "Emotional pain is the experience of ...perceived threat or damage to our emotional self, the 'sense' of who we are, and our psychological self. But then, like physical pain, we want to understand it because we want the pain to go away. This is where suffering can start. We create a story about the meaning of emotional pain. The story is inherently subjective." And we have the power to revise it. https://livingsystems.ca/emotional-pain-and-suffering/#:~:text=Emotional%20pain%20is%20the%20experience,is%20where%20suffering%20can%20start.

Suffering Results From Wanting Things To Be Different

You have heard the maxim, "The only constant is change." You must grieve the loss when something ends, but understanding that endings are new beginnings lessens the pain. "...As much as we want to hold onto the things, people, and feelings we like, we'll always have to deal with separation and loss. There's suffering any time we want things to be different than they are." All the ideas and quotes in the rest of this chapter are from the Recovery Dharma Book, which you can access for free at this website. https://recoverydharma.org/book/

The Intersection of Addiction, Recovery, and Mental Health

Where addiction and mental health meet, there is an intricate interplay of pain, suffering, and the quest for relief. At the core of this struggle lies a dangerous risk – the risk of suicide. In this context, the ancient wisdom of the Four Noble Truths, the Eightfold Path, and the transformative principles of Recovery Dharma offer a beacon of hope, guiding you toward a life of balance, understanding, and peace.

Understanding the Link between Addiction and Suicide

Before delving into the therapeutic applications of Recovery Dharma and the Eightfold Path, it's imperative to understand the link between addiction and suicide. Addiction, often a maladaptive response to trauma or emotional pain, leads to a cycle of despair and hopelessness. This despair, compounded by the neurological and social consequences of substance abuse, significantly heightens the risk of suicide.

Recovery Dharma: A Holistic Approach

Recovery Dharma emerges as a groundbreaking approach, merging Buddhist philosophy with modern recovery methods. It focuses on understanding the nature of suffering, the cause of suffering, and the path leading out of suffering – aligning seamlessly with the Four Noble Truths of Buddhism. In addressing addiction, Recovery Dharma doesn't merely seek to treat the symptoms; it aims to transform the root causes of suffering by realizing you can modify those stories causing the suffering.

Applying the Four Noble Truths in Addiction Recovery and Suicide Prevention

The Four Noble Truths, the cornerstone of Buddhist teachings, offer profound insights into the nature of suffering and the path to liberation. When applied to addiction recovery and suicide prevention, these truths provide a framework for understanding the deep-rooted causes of suffering and charting a course toward healing and resilience.

The First Noble Truth: The Truth of Suffering (Dukkha)

"Our senses (which the Buddha understood to include not just hearing, seeing, smelling, tasting, and touch but also thinking) are unreliable (impersonal) and temporary (impermanent), which means that the way we experience and make sense of the world is constantly changing. We suffer because we keep expecting these temporary experiences to satisfy our craving for pleasure or to avoid pain."

The Reality of Suffering

- **Trauma and attachment injuries:** They are not our fault, but healing from them is our "responsibility" and "right." "Developing understanding and compassion toward (how) trauma affects our reactions to events or circumstances now is an important part of that healing."

- **Addiction as Suffering**: Addiction is a form of suffering. It's not merely a series of poor choices or a moral failing; it's a manifestation of more profound pain and dissatisfaction with life.

- **Comprehending the Scope**: Suffering extends beyond physical or mental anguish; it includes the subtler aspects of dissatisfaction, uncertainty, and impermanence that characterize human existence.

- **Relation to Suicide Risk**: The deep suffering caused by addiction often leads to feelings of hopelessness and despair, which can escalate to suicidal ideation.

The Second Noble Truth: The Truth of the Cause of Suffering (Samudaya)

"Addiction creates a hope that both pleasure and escape can be permanent. We repeatedly suffer because substances or behaviors can only temporarily relieve our pain, unhappiness, and lost or damaged sense of self..."

Identifying the Roots of Addiction and Despair

- **Craving and Attachment**: At the heart of suffering is craving – for pleasure, avoidance of discomfort, and permanence in an impermanent world. In addiction, this craving manifests as a compulsive need for substances or behaviors that provide temporary relief.

- **Understanding the Cycle**: Recognizing how addictive behaviors are attempts to escape suffering, yet ironically, they perpetuate more suffering.

- **Addressing Underlying Issues**: Identifying and addressing underlying issues such as trauma, mental health disorders, or emotional pain that fuel addictive behaviors and suicidal thoughts.

The Third Noble Truth: The Truth of the End of Suffering (Nirodha)

"Realize that all experiences are temporary by nature and that we can appreciate what is exactly as it is and end our craving for something different... which creates our suffering. We choose what we think, say, and do. We are entirely responsible for our happiness, and we can reduce our suffering by simply accepting what is (precisely) as it is, right here, right now."

Envisioning a Path to Liberation

- **Hope and Possibility**: The realization that it's possible to end suffering. For someone struggling with addiction and suicidal thoughts, this truth instills hope that recovery and peace of mind are attainable.

- **Breaking the Cycle**: Understanding that by letting go of cravings and attachments, individuals can break the cycle of addiction and the resultant risk of suicide.

The Fourth Noble Truth: The Truth of the Path That Leads to the End of Suffering (Magga)

"The Buddha taught that by living ethically, practicing meditation, and developing wisdom and compassion, we can end the suffering we create by resisting, running from, and misunderstanding reality."

The Eightfold Path: A Framework for Healing

The Eightfold Path, central to Buddhist teachings, offers a practical framework for overcoming addiction and reducing suicide risk. This path includes:

1. **Wise Understanding**: Living without clinging, attachment, or craving because you understand life's impermanence and unsatisfactory nature and how your actions contribute to your suffering or happiness.

2. **Wise Intent**: Cultivating intentions of renunciation, goodwill, and harmlessness. This step involves a commitment to change and the development of a compassionate attitude towards yourself and others.

3. **Wise Speech**: Engaging in truthful, positive, and helpful communication. This practice builds a support system and reduces the isolation we often experience in addiction.

4. **Wise Action**: Committing to ethical conduct includes abstaining from substances and behaviors that harm yourself or others. Of

course, you can't stop eating or using electronics, but you can set limits.

5. **Wise Livelihood**: Choosing a way of life that is ethical, responsible, and harmonious, avoiding occupations or activities that contribute to addiction.

6. **Wise Effort**: Cultivating positive states of mind, replacing harmful thoughts and behaviors with beneficial ones.

7. **Wise Mindfulness**: Developing awareness of one's thoughts, feelings, and bodily sensations in the present moment, which is particularly effective in managing cravings and emotional turmoil.

8. **Wise Concentration**: Practicing meditation to develop deeper insight and tranquility, strengthening the mind's ability to cope with stress and triggers.

Walking the Eightfold Path

- **Implementing Practical Steps**: The Eightfold Path offers practical steps for overcoming addiction and reducing the risk of suicide.

- **Holistic Approach**: Emphasizing the importance of a comprehensive approach that includes ethical living, mental discipline, and wisdom.

- **Continuous Practice**: Recognize that the path is not a quick fix but a lifelong journey of growth and discovery.

- **The Role of Meditation and Mindfulness**

Mindfulness and meditation are central to the Eightfold Path and Recovery Dharma. These practices enhance self-awareness and emotional regulation, central components in managing addiction and suicidal ideation. By staying grounded in the present moment, you better equip yourself to handle cravings and emotional distress without resorting to substance use or self-harm.

Group Support and Community

A vital component of Recovery Dharma is its emphasis on community and group support. Sharing experiences and insights within a group setting creates a sense of connection and mutual understanding, counteracting the isolation that often accompanies addiction and suicidal thoughts.

Understanding and Liberation

The Four Noble Truths illuminate your understanding, healing, and liberation. Adopting these truths allows you to comprehend your suffering and live the eightfold path with renewed purpose and peace. Meditation, mindfulness, and attending support groups will lend you purpose and belonging, mitigating despair and hopelessness. The recovery dharma is grounded in ancient wisdom and offers a powerful testament to the resilience of the human spirit and the potential for transformation and renewal.

The ninth secret for you is to incorporate the Recovery Dharma, Four Noble Truths, and Eightfold Path into your addiction treatment to lessen your suicide risk. Again, all the ideas and quotes from this chapter are from the Recovery Dharma Book, which you can access for free on this website. https://recoverydharma.org/book/

Other Addictions

"Jon," I said, "People don't realize that overeating, or suicide ideation, or overdoing work or sports can be addictions." "Yeah," replied Jon, "I think I have been a workaholic sometimes and a food addict at other times. But my wife left me because she decided she wanted to have sex with a woman instead of me. I am not sure what to do with that one, so I suppose I have become a workaholic once again. I just have to keep working so I don't think about it."

Chapter 11
Healthy Relationships With Others

Lost in the Past

"You know, Mom," observed Eve. "My body is really shaky right now. I feel hot and sweaty from the sun in this car and overwhelmed by what you are sharing right now. I love you so much, but I am not a therapist. I know you miss Terry, and I can't even imagine all the things you have been through, but I am afraid you might miss this time right now because you are so focused on your loss in the past."

Get Therapy

"Wow," I replied, "You are so wise, even at twenty-one. Thanks for pulling me out of this funk. I guess I want to share my grief with someone." Eve added, "That's understandable, but no one can handle when you emotionally bleed all over them. That's why there are therapists."

The tenth secret for you is to engage in healthy relationships with others to lower your suicide risk. Engaging in healthy relationships with others requires understanding the difference between healthy and unhealthy and nurturing those connections that are emotionally supportive and empowering for you.

Relationship Factors

Relationship factors were one of the four risk factors mentioned in the chapter on Why Suicide? One-Fifth of Suicide Deaths Linked to Relationship Problems. "One in five deaths by suicide is related to problems with current or former intimate partners such as divorce, separation, romantic breakups, conflicts, and intimate partner violence, a study in the American Journal of Preventive Medicine has found." https://psychiatryonline.org/doi/full/10.1176/appi.pn.2023.06.6.7

How Do You Engage in Healthy Relationships With Others?

In this chapter, I want to emphasize that having a healthy relationship with others always begins with having a healthy relationship with yourself. Also, as you interact with others, there are distinctive patterns to recognize, warning signs of dysfunctional relationships and communication skills you can learn to enhance your ability to connect with honesty and integrity.

Focus On Changing Yourself

Unfortunately, you can never control anyone outside yourself, so trying to change anyone else is futile. Fortunately, you change your life by altering your physical/emotional state and vibrational energy and expanding your identity to an improved version of yourself through actions that improve your self-esteem because you have done something difficult for yourself. You have pushed through and earned self-respect!

Quality of Relationships

"The quality of your relationships determines the quality of your life." —Tony Robbins.

In the eighth secret, you learned that the most important relationship to nurture is the one with yourself because as you get healthier, you attract healthier people. You will leave dysfunctional relationships, or they will fade out of your life when you set firm boundaries and no longer let others manipulate you.

Dysfunctional Relationships Resulting From Early Attachment Disorders

It's not your fault your early caregivers weren't healthy, but it is your right and responsibility to heal. One of life's most challenging experiences is dealing with dysfunctional relationships with family, friends, romantic partners, or in professional settings. That is why anonymous people organically formed various twelve-step groups— to help one another handle dysfunctional relationships.

Distinct Patterns

Dysfunctional relationships have distinct patterns of unhealthy behavior and interaction. Understanding and identifying them will aid in unearthing appropriate solutions or interventions. Here are some of the most prevalent:

1. Codependent Relationships: In a codependent relationship, one partner typically sacrifices their needs and well-being to satisfy the other. This dynamic often involves one person enabling another's addiction, poor mental health, immaturity, irresponsibility, or underachievement.

2. Controlling Relationships: One partner dominates the other through manipulation, intimidation, or violence. This control can manifest in dictating who their partner can see, what they can do, or how they should think and feel.

3. Abusive Relationships: Characteristics of these relationships are physical, emotional, sexual, or psychological abuse. Abusive behavior includes insults, threats, isolation, and physical violence. The abuse can be overt or subtle, but it consistently undermines the victim's sense of self-worth and safety.

4. Avoidant/Dependent Relationships: One partner is emotionally distant and avoids intimacy, while the other partner craves closeness and becomes overly dependent. This imbalance creates a push-pull dynamic that is stressful and unsatisfying for both parties.

5. Conflict-Avoidant Relationships: In these relationships, partners avoid conflict at all costs. While this might seem peaceful, it often leads to unresolved issues, resentment, and a lack of genuine emotional connection.

6. Competitive/Combative Relationships: Constant competition or arguments mark these relationships. Partners may compete for attention, success, or control, often leading to a toxic cycle of one-upmanship.

7. Enmeshed Relationships: Boundaries are blurred or nonexistent in enmeshed relationships. Individuals lose their sense of self and independence, often feeling responsible for their partner's emotions and well-being, leading to a loss of personal identity.

8. Passive-Aggressive Relationships: Communication in these relationships is indirect and manipulative. One or both partners may express their negative feelings subtly rather than openly addressing issues, leading to a lack of trust and open communication.

9. Narcissistic Relationships: One partner, typically a narcissist, dominates these relationships. They lack empathy, are often preoccupied with their own needs and accomplishments, and can be emotionally abusive.

10. Parent-Child Dynamics in Adult Relationships: These relationships feature an unhealthy parent-child dynamic where one partner assumes a superior, caretaking role and the other a submissive, child-like role. This dynamic hinders the development of a mature, equal partnership.

11. The Savior Complex: One partner feels compelled to "save" the other, often attracting partners who are perceived to need fixing. This rescuing can create an imbalanced relationship where one person has more power and control.

12. The Silent Relationship: Communication is minimal in these relationships, and partners may live parallel lives with little interaction. Emotional connection and intimacy are often lacking.

13. Cyclical Relationships: Characterized by repetitive breakups and reconciliations, these relationships create a confusing cycle that emotionally exhausts both partners and prevents them from moving forward.

14. Substance Dependent Relationships: These revolve around one or both partners' substance misuse, which often takes precedence over the relationship's health, leading to neglect, abuse, and dysfunction.

Addressing the Underlying Issues

Identifying these patterns in a relationship is the first step toward addressing the underlying issues. While you can improve some dysfunctional relationships with counseling, twelve-step groups, and a genuine willingness to change, in others, particularly those in toxic or abusive relationships with a severe imbalance, it becomes necessary to consider leaving the relationship for your safety and well-being. It's crucial to approach these situations with self-compassion and, where required, seek support from friends, family, or professionals.

Red Flags

Notice the Red Flags: Pay attention to feelings of constant distress, anxiety, resentment, or feeling belittled, not taken seriously, lack of intimacy (not just sexual), walking on eggshells because of the power imbalance, frequent blaming instead of taking responsibility, avoiding the other person, codependent feelings like you can't exist without the other person, in a relationship because abuse can be emotional, physical, sexual, or psychological. Regular conflicts, lack of support, and controlling behaviors are vital indicators of a toxic relationship.

Emotional Abuse

Accusations of cheating, gaslighting, isolating the other from family and friends, withholding attention and affection as punishment, continuous criticism, trivializing concerns, name-calling, and verbal abuse like using words to attack, dominate, ridicule, manipulate, or degrade the other person.
https://www.blakepsychology.com/2022/03/what-are-the-signs-of-a-dysfunctional-relationship/#:~:text=The%20word%20%E2%80%9Cdysfunctional%E2%80%9D%20or%20%E2%80%9C,bringing%20you%20joy%20and%20support.

Safety Plan For Leaving

If you decide to leave, it is essential to have a safety plan for leaving if you are in danger, just as you have a plan for crisis moments in suicidal ideation. This plan may involve contacting support services, finding a safe stay, and understanding legal rights. See my Escaping Domestic Violence: A Survivor's Truth book for resources.

Counseling can be a valuable tool in dealing with dysfunctional relationships. It provides a neutral ground to discuss issues and professional guidance in navigating complex emotions and situations. Personal therapy can help understand one's role in the relationship dynamics and develop strategies to cope with or improve the situation. In cases where both parties are willing to work on the relationship, couple or family therapy can effectively resolve conflicts and improve communication.

Self-Care and Support Systems

While dealing with dysfunctional relationships, self-care becomes even more crucial. Build a support network with friends, family or support groups to lean on for emotional support and practical advice. Engaging in activities that promote well-being, like exercise, hobbies, and relaxation techniques, can reduce stress and improve mood.

Open and honest communication is the cornerstone of resolving issues in any relationship. It involves expressing feelings without blame and actively listening to the other person's perspective. Establishing clear boundaries with respectful but firm communication is essential. They help define acceptable behavior and what is not, thus protecting your emotional health.

SEW Technique

Dr. Julia Coldwell explains that no one wants to be controlled. When one person in a relationship tries to control the other, the "initial placation.. inevitably turns into resistance and resentment." Her technique is "telling the unarguable truth through SEW.

Begin With Sensations

Because our experiences are subjective, tuning into your bodily sensations, which are unarguable, you exhibit your underlying beliefs, which are arguable. Starting with your sensations focuses on the issue instead of blaming or projecting.

Emotions

Following sensations leads you to your emotions. For example, the tension in the jaw, neck, and shoulders shows anger because you are not getting what you want or you are getting something you don't want. A tight throat or heavy chest signifies sadness from loss. Stomach turmoil displays fear.

Want

Expressing the heightened awareness of your sensations and letting your emotions flow through will let you voice what you genuinely want. Your body has the answers, but it'll need time to convey them unarguably. Both people need turns verbalizing their initial situation and reactions to the other's truth, always using the SEW process. This communication tool uses honesty and boundaries and can avert arguments. https://www.patheos.com/blogs/evolutionarypower/archives/2078

Healing and Moving Forward

Whether the resolution involves mending or ending the relationship, healing from its impact takes time.

Acceptance and Forgiveness: This involves accepting what has happened and, where possible, forgiving (not necessarily reconciling) to let go of anger and resentment. Forgiveness is more about your own peace than condoning or excusing the other person's behavior.

Learning from Experience: Reflect on the relationship to understand what went wrong and how similar situations can be avoided or handled better in the future.

Rebuilding Self-Esteem: Dysfunctional relationships often diminish your self-esteem. Engaging in activities that reinforce self-worth and completing challenging things can help restore confidence.

Self-Awareness, Communication, Professional Help, Self-Care

Dealing with dysfunctional relationships is a complex and often painful process. It requires a combination of self-awareness, communication, professional help, and self-care. Utilizing the SEW technique forges honest communication with proper boundaries and can diminish misunderstandings. Each situation is unique, and the path to resolution varies. The most important thing is to prioritize your safety and emotional well-being.

Engage in Healthy Relationships

By addressing these issues head-on and making informed decisions, you can emerge more robust and resilient from dysfunctional relationships. Your immediate safety and professional assistance are paramount in situations of abuse. Healing is a personal journey; seeking help and taking the time to recover and rebuild is okay so that you can engage in healthy relationships. The tenth secret for you is to engage in healthy relationships with others to lower your suicide risk.

Continued Conversation With Eve

"Gotcha," I responded. Eve ended, "Well, I want you to be happy, and I don't want you to feel like you can't express yourself, Mom, but let's enjoy this time together, alright? I want to find this hiking trail my friend recommended here in Tucson. Sound good?" "Hey Eve, you just used the SEW method of communication that I have been learning about: sensations, emotions, and wants... so cool. Yeah, honey, let's go find the trail," I said as I opened the car door.

Chapter 12 Community and Connection

I Can't Do it Anymore

"Hello, Mija, what's up?" asked my mom on the other end of the telephone line. "I just can't do it anymore," I sobbed. "I have tried everything: medication, counseling, and leaving my abusive husband, but I can't stop the pain. He'll never change, and I will never be able to protect my children."

Suicide Affects Your Children

"I know, honey. I understand. Anyone in your situation would feel the same way. You have wrestled with this for years. No one could blame you," Mom sighed. "But you do know how much it affects your children, right? Will it be Josh, Ben, or Miriam that follows your example? Which one of them killing themselves would be okay with you?"

They Deserve Happiness

I burst into deeper sobs, "But they are good," I said. "They deserve to live happy, healthy lives!" Mom replied, "So do you, Mija. You are good, too, and who will help them if you aren't there? Their violent dad?"

The eleventh secret for you is to take action personally, as a family, and as a community because you can make a difference! Suicide affects everyone. In our greater community, when Robin Williams killed himself, some part of me died. He had kept me laughing through decades of trauma. In my family, when my sister killed herself, my heart dropped. When I had taken bottles of pills, my mom reminded me of my children's trauma, PTSD, anxiety, or depression, leading to their suicides if I ended my life, so Emergency Medical Technicians (EMTs) got me to the hospital in time to pump my stomach again.

Personal Tragedy

Suicide is often the culmination of an intense and seemingly impossible struggle with mental health issues, such as depression, anxiety, or other disorders, unaddressed childhood trauma, chronic pain, job or financial loss, legal problems, violence, or substance abuse. This personal tragedy represents a moment of profound hopelessness and pain.

Suicide's Lie

Suicide's lie is that it will end that suffering. It doesn't— not for yourself or anyone that knows you. My near-death experience revealed that we carry the same vibrational energy and consciousness into the afterlife, so this life is the time to lift your vibrations and rebuild yourself anew. When you connect to the heartbeat and LOVE of the Universe, our greater community, through your heart portal, you emerge as an enlarged being.

Problems

Remember that suffering results from wanting things to be different than they are because we think we aren't supposed to have problems. That is the problem. Challenges are the process of growth and our love evolution. Letting go of the old belief that you aren't supposed to have obstacles is an inner death so that the flowering, deeper, more authentic you is born.

Missed Magical Relationship

Killing yourself just limits your opportunity to have more joy. When I met Terry, the "love of my life," I remember realizing that if I had been successful in my previous suicide attempts, I would have missed the nine pleasurable, fun, and nurturing years with him. I was so grateful for our magical relationship!

Missed Joy of Children

Then I realized that had I taken my life when I was younger, I would have missed my greatest joy of having my children! I felt fortunate that I had failed to take my life so I could enjoy my kids and grandkids and still have the potential to grow, overcome challenges, heal, and find joy again.

Loved Ones

Loved ones, whether life partners, family, friends, or even communities, are devastated as they grapple with overwhelming grief, unanswered questions, and often feelings of guilt or anger when you kill yourself. The sudden and violent nature of suicide can be particularly traumatizing, leaving deep emotional scars, so the pain doesn't disappear; you merely transfer it to the survivors.

Family History of Suicide

A family history of suicide can increase the risk of suicidal thoughts for survivors, which may compound the potential genetic predisposition to mental health issues and the traumatic impact of a family member's suicide. As a surviving family member, you must understand they "didn't do it because you didn't love them enough." Let the guilt go.

Open Conversations: It's important to talk openly about mental health and the family's history. This openness can remove the stigma and make it easier to seek help when needed.

Mental Health Education: It is crucial to educate the family on the signs of mental distress and the resources available for help. This awareness can help in early intervention and prevention.

Individual Therapy: Those with a family history of suicide should consider regular therapy sessions, even if they currently do not have suicidal thoughts. This preemptive approach can provide them with coping strategies and a safe space to discuss issues as they arise.

Community Loss

Suicide impacts communities through loss, grief, and mourning as well. Each casualty resonates through schools, workplaces, neighborhoods, countries, and societies, leaving a void that is felt by many. In addition, the "suicide contagion effect" can increase the risk of further suicides and lead to a heightened sense of vulnerability with a greater need for careful, compassionate community support and mental health resources.

Community and Connection

Social support plays a critical role in mental health and well-being. Communities act as safety nets, creating a solid emotional support network that provides connection, belonging, purpose, practical help, and security, alleviating hopelessness and despair. This support system can take many forms, including family, friends, co-workers, or members of social groups or clubs. Volunteering is another excellent way for individuals to feel connected and valued in their community.

Reducing Stigma through Openness and Education

Communities that foster openness about mental health challenges help in reducing the stigma associated with them. Education and awareness initiatives within communities can encourage more people to seek help and share their experiences without fear of judgment. Support groups are the perfect vehicle for this, and many resources to find the right one for you are in the chapter on Prevention.

Reaching Out and Being Vulnerable

Building supportive relationships often requires taking the first step to reach out and be vulnerable. It may seem inconceivable to initiate conversation, but sharing your struggles with trusted individuals can open the door to deeper connections and support. Regular participation can also strengthen those ties and provide a consistent sense of community. You deserve to feel supported and loved!

Being a Supportive Community Member

Supportive relationships are a two-way street. Being there for others in their time of need and offering a listening ear or practical help can strengthen your relationships and build a more resilient community. It requires sincere effort, vulnerability, and a commitment to community involvement. Whether face-to-face interactions or digital platforms, these contacts can offer kinship, compassion, and support during crises and pave the way for healing and hope.

Communities Can Tackle Bullying and Violence

Bullying and violence can leave deep emotional scars, often contributing to suicidal thoughts. The first step in overcoming this is recognizing the signs of bullying: withdrawal, unexplained injuries, or a sudden drop in self-esteem. Once identified, creating a safe and supportive environment for the victim is essential. Please encourage them to construct a new identity where they won't allow others to cross their boundaries anymore.

Intervention Strategies: Schools and workplaces must implement anti-bullying policies and programs. For those already affected, counseling and support groups can provide a safe space to discuss experiences and emotions. Additionally, teaching coping mechanisms like resilience training can empower victims to handle future conflicts better.

Community Support: Building a community support system is vital. This support system can include friends, family, teachers, or co-workers who know the situation and can offer emotional support. In severe cases, law enforcement or legal action might be necessary to ensure the individual's safety. We must elect leaders who will enforce laws against child sexual slavery and the like.

Social Isolation

Social isolation can significantly contribute to suicidal thoughts. This isolation could be due to various factors, including mental health issues, physical disabilities, or social anxieties. Therapists specializing in social skills training can assist in building confidence in social settings. According to experts, cognitive behavioral therapy (CBT) is particularly effective in changing negative thought patterns that contribute to social isolation.

Online Connections

Technology plays a crucial role in maintaining connections in today's digital age. Online communities, support groups, therapists, video calls, and social media can help people stay connected and reduce loneliness, especially those who are physically isolated or have mobility issues. Many online resources are listed in the chapter on prevention, and always remember 988 in crisis moments.

Managing Relationship Loss

The end of a significant relationship, whether it be a romantic breakup, a friendship ending, or a death, can be a trigger for suicidal thoughts. Professional grief counseling and grief support groups where you can share your experiences with others who have faced similar situations can be beneficial and provide a structured way to process the loss. Attending a grief group benefited my youngest daughter, Eve, and me after Terry died.

Rebuilding Self-Identity and Staying Connected

Rebuilding self-identity and staying connected are vital as you rediscover who you are outside the lost relationship. Exploring hobbies, interests, and personal goals can help rebuild a sense of self and purpose while staying connected with family and friends, who provide a support network and avert loneliness during this vulnerable time. I am still in that process.

Remembering and Honoring the Deceased

Finding ways to remember and honor the deceased can aid healing. These ways might involve creating a memorial, writing letters to them, or participating in activities they enjoyed doing while they were with you. These acts can keep their memory alive and provide a sense of closure. We often speak of things Terry taught us because he was so wise and funny! Keeping loved ones in our hearts helps avert the loneliness of them being physically gone.

Taking Care of Yourself

It's easy to neglect your well-being amid grief. However, caring for your physical and mental health is essential for healing. Ensure you get enough rest, eat well, and engage in activities that bring you comfort and relaxation.

Suicide Doesn't Stop the Pain

Suicide affects everyone. It is a tragedy because the person misses out on any future opportunities to experience growth and joy. It is a dirty deception that suicide will end the torment. It doesn't. That is why I wrote this book to shred suicide's lie: it doesn't stop the suffering. Your vibration and consciousness follow you into the afterlife, and you also transfer your misery to your surviving loved ones.

What Families and Communities Can Do

If you are a surviving family member of suicide, it's necessary to have frank discussions about mental health and therapy in your family to prevent more trauma. Communities can provide connection to combat loneliness (in-person or online), foster openness and education, provide bullying intervention, offer grief support as you rebuild your identity, honor the deceased, remember to take care of yourself and enlist valuable emotional support.

Open to Hope

Take action. Keep your personal safety plan near. Be resourceful, get therapy or commit to a support group, even if online groups are all you can muster right now. With a support system, proper treatment, and incorporating habits that raise your vital energy, you can regain hope, relieve misery, and again feel joy. You are meant to feel deep inner peace and satisfaction. You deserve to be happy! Open to hope. And remember that you are not alone—

The eleventh secret for you is to take action personally, as a family, and as a community because you can make a difference! For those extending emotional support, as friends and family with a listening ear, who encourage professional help, stay involved, and advocate for change in your community, you can help prevent the tragedy of suicide from happening to someone else. You are making a difference! You made a difference for me. I am still alive to write this book because of YOU. Thank you for being my beacon of hope!

Keep Living

"Okay, mom. I have to keep on living for my kids. Thank you for reminding me how my suicide would affect my kids. Will you call the ambulance to pick me up because the pills are kicking in, and I can't see the numbers on my phone anymore?" I asked. She called the ambulance, and I survived. Shred suicide's lie and let hope live in you as it is in me. YOU deserve to live happily!

Chapter 13
Quick Recap of the 11SecretsForYou:

The first secret for You is to understand WHY someone might want to commit suicide. Then, you have an idea where to start to help them prevent it and support them emotionally.

The second secret for You is to realize that suicide will not provide the relief sought because we carry the same vibrational energy and consciousness into the afterlife.

The third secret for You is recognizing warning signs and using empathic communication.

The fourth secret for You is to know what to expect when you contact 988 and how to help on social media.

The fifth secret for You is creating and implementing a safety plan for crisis moments.

The sixth secret for You is to locate a longer-term therapist, use online resources, watch videos, and find the right support group to help you avoid crises.

The seventh secret for You is prioritizing caring for your body and mind so that you can thrive after trauma.

The eighth secret for You is to create a healthy relationship with yourself to reduce your suicide risk.

The ninth secret for You is to incorporate the Recovery Dharma, Four Noble Truths, and Eightfold Path into your addiction treatment to lessen your suicide risk.

The tenth secret for You is to engage in healthy relationships with others to lower your suicide risk.

The eleventh secret for You is to take action personally, as a family, and as a community because you can make a difference!

Chapter 14
Works Cited:

988 Suicide & Crisis Lifeline. (n.d.-a). *988 suicide & crisis lifeline.* 988 Suicide & Crisis Lifeline, Retrieved (January 31, 2024) from https://988lifeline.org/

988 Suicide & Crisis Lifeline. (n.d.-c). *988 suicide & crisis lifeline.* 988 Suicide & Crisis Lifeline, Retrieved (January 31, 2024) from https://988lifeline.org/chat/

988 Suicide & Crisis Lifeline. *American Indian, Alaska natives, indigenous peoples.* 988 Lifeline. (n.d.-b). Retrieved May 29, 2026) from https://988lifeline.org/help-yourself/americanindian-alaskanatives-indigenouspeoples/

988 Suicide & Crisis Lifeline. (n.d.-c). *Help someone else.* 988 Suicide & Crisis Lifeline. https://988lifeline.org/help-someone-else/

988 Suicide & Crisis Lifeline. (n.d.-d). *Help yourself.* 988 Suicide & Crisis Lifeline, Retrieved (January 31, 2024) from https://988lifeline.org/help-yourself/

988 Suicide & Crisis Lifeline. (n.d.-e). *Stories of hope and recovery.* 988 Suicide & Crisis Lifeline, Retrieved (January 31, 2024) from https://988lifeline.org/stories/

988 Suicide & Crisis Lifeline. (n.d.-f). *Support on social media.* 988 Suicide & Crisis Lifeline, Retrieved (January 31, 2024) from https://988lifeline.org/help-someone-else/safety-and-support-on-social-media/

Alcoholics Anonymous. (n.d.). *The twelve steps.* Alcoholics Anonymous, Retrieved (February 2, 2024) from https://www.aa.org/the-twelve-steps

Al-Anon. (n.d.). *The twelve steps.* Al-Anon. Retrieved (February 2, 2024) from https://al-anon.org/for-members/the-legacies/the-twelve-steps/

Ankrom, S. (2023, January 27). *Deep breathing exercises to reduce anxiety*. Verywell Mind, Retrieved (January 31, 2024) from https://www.verywellmind.com/abdominal-breathing-2584115

Beer-Becker, D. (2023, December 15). *What are the signs of a dysfunctional relationship?*. Blake Psychology, Retrieved (January 31, 2024) from https://www.blakepsychology.com/2022/03/what-are-the-signs-of-a-dysfunctional-relationship/#:~:text=The%20word%20%E2%80%9Cdysfunctional%E2%80%9D%20or%20%E2%80%9C,bringing%20you%20joy%20and%20support.

Benoit, D. (2004, October). *Infant-parent attachment: Definition, types, antecedents, measurement and outcome*. Paediatrics & child health, Retrieved (January 31, 2024) from https://www.ncbi.nlm.nih.gov/pmc/articles/PMC2724160/#:~:text=Of%20the%20four%20patterns%20of,2,18%E2%80%9324

Centers for Disease Control and Prevention. (2025, March 26). *Facts about suicide*. Centers for Disease Control and Prevention, Retrieved (May 29, 2026) from https://www.cdc.gov/suicide/facts/data.html

Chi, C. (n.d.). *The David Hawkins Scale (navigating emotional states)*. r/mentalhealth, Retrieved (January 31, 2024) from https://www.reddit.com/r/mentalhealth/comments/wd6snu/the_david_hawkins_scale_navigating_emotional/?rdt=55610

Clark, C. (2021, September 12). *EMDR safe place bilateral relaxation meditation with therapist Carmel Clark*. YouTube, Retrieved (January 31, 2024) from https://www.youtube.com/watch?v=IQI82AvvWNI

Colwell, J. (2026). *S.E.W.-ing your way out of power struggle | Julie Colwell*. patheos.com/Evolutionary Power, Retrieved (May 27, 2026) from https://www.patheos.com/blogs/evolutionarypower/archives/2078

D 'Arrigo, T. (2023, May 22). *One-fifth of suicide deaths linked to relationship problems | psychiatric news*. Psychiatric News, Retrieved (May 27, 2026) from https://psychiatryonline.org/doi/full/10.1176/appi.pn.2023.06.6.7

Emotions anonymous 12 step program of recovery. Emotions Anonymous. (2026), Retrieved May 29, 2026) from https://emotionsanonymous.org/

Fraga, J., Caplan, E., (2024, January 25). *9 affordable therapy options for 2024*. Healthline, Retrieved (January 31, 2024) from https://www.healthline.com/health/therapy-for-every-budget#A-quick-look-at-the-best-affordable-therapy-resources

Franz, P., & Jayson , S. (2023, November 28). *Suicide warning signs in older adults*. AARP, Retrieved (May 29, 2026) from https://www.aarp.org/health/healthy-living/suicides-rising-among-older-men/

Global Suicide Hotline Resources. (n.d.). *Global suicide hotline resources: Whatsapp help center*. Global Suicide Hotline Resources | WhatsApp Help Center, Retrieved (January 31, 2024) from https://faq.whatsapp.com/1417269125743673/?locale=en_US

Goltzman, J. (2022, February 28). *6 best online depression support groups for 2022*. Healthline, Retrieved (January 31, 2024) from https://www.healthline.com/health/mental-health/online-depression-support-groups#A-quick-look-at-the-best-online-support-groups-for-depression

Graham, L. (2020, September 7). *The triangle of victim, rescuer, persecutor - what it is and how to get out*, Retrieved (January 31, 2024) from https://lindagraham-mft.net/triangle-victim-rescuer-persecutor-get/

International Association for Suicide Prevention. (2023a, May 23). *Global suicide statistics*. IASP, Retrieved (January 31, 2024) from https://www.iasp.info/wspd/references/#:~:text=An%20estimated%20703%20000%20people%20die%20by%20suicide%20worldwide%20each%20year.&text=Over%20one%20in%20every%20100,was%20the%20result%20of%20suicide.&text=The%20global%20suicide%20rate%20is,high%20among%20men%20than%20women.&text=Over%20half%20(58%25)%20of,age%20of%2050%20years%20old.

International Association for Suicide Prevention. (2023b, August 18). *Suicidal crisis support.* IASP, Retrieved (January 31, 2024) from https://www.iasp.info/suicidalthoughts/

Living Systems Counselling. (2022, August 15). *Emotional pain and suffering are different.* Living Systems Counselling, Retrieved (January 31, 2024) from https://livingsystems.ca/emotional-pain-and-suffering/#:~:text=Emotional%20pain%20is%20the%20experience,is%20where%20suffering%20can%20start.

McDonnell, W. (1983, June 9). *Analysis and Assessment of Gateway Process.* Central Intelligence Agency, Retrieved (May 30, 2026) from https://www.cia.gov/readingroom/docs/cia-rdp96-00788r001700210016-5.pdf

Mcleod, S. (2024, January 24). *Maslow's hierarchy of needs.* Simply Psychology, Retrieved (January 31, 2024) from https://www.simplypsychology.org/maslow.html#The-expanded-hierarchy-of-needs

McTaggart, Lynne. *The Field.* Harper Collins, 13 Oct. 2009.

Mieke, meditate. (2023, August 27). *EMDR | Visual Meditation | Self-administered | healing.* YouTube, Retrieved (January 31, 2024) from https://www.youtube.com/watch?v=DheesiCVbK8

National Institute of Mental Health. (2023, May 22). *Youth suicide rates increased during the covid-19 pandemic,* Retrieved (May 29, 2026) from https://www.nimh.nih.gov/news/science-updates/2023/youth-suicide-rates-increased-during-the-covid-19-pandemic

Pasterski, M. (2020, August 25). *Types of parts in IFS,* Retrieved (January 31, 2024) from https://pasterski.com/2019/11/types-of-parts-in-ifs/

Recovery Dharma Global. (2024, January 15). *Book • recovery dharma.* Recovery Dharma, Retrieved (January 31, 2024) from https://recoverydharma.org/book/

Richburg, J. (2019, December 1). *10-Minute Body Scan Meditation.* YouTube, Retrieved (January 31, 2024) from https://www.youtube.com/watch?v=uqtlqCKjkuc

Robbins, T. (2023). *Tony Robbins Priming Exercise.* YouTube, Retrieved (May 30, 2026) from https://www.youtube.com/watch?v=m2ix1iAbbfc

Robinson, L. (2024, January 8). *Attachment styles and how they affect adult relationships.* HelpGuide.org, Retrieved (January 31, 2024) from https://www.helpguide.org/articles/relationships-communication/attachment-and-adult-relationships.htm#:~:text=Disorganized%20attachment-,Secure%20attachment%20style:%20what%20it%20looks%20like,thrive%20in%20close,%20meaningful%20relationships.

Rooms, I. T. (2026). *Online recovery community, live addiction meetings &12 step meetings online.* IN THE ROOMS. https://www.intherooms.com/home/category/community-and-meetings/

Sanford, M. *Adaptive yoga videos: The MBS Online Video Hub.* Mind Body Solutions. (2023, November 8). https://www.mindbodysolutions.org/video-hub/

Stanborough, R. J. (2020, November 13). *What is vibrational energy? definition, benefits & more.* Healthline, Retrieved (January 31, 2024) from https://www.healthline.com/health/vibrational-energy#what-we-know

Substance Abuse and Mental Health Services Administration. (2010, April). *To live to see the Great Day that dawns: Preventing suicide by American Indian and Alaska native youth and young adults.* To Live To See the Great Day That Dawns: Preventing Suicide by American Indian and Alaska Native Youth and Young Adults | SAMHSA Publications and Digital Products, Retrieved (January 31, 2024) from https://store.samhsa.gov/product/to-live-to-see-the-great-day-that-dawns-preventing-suicide-american-indian-alaska-native-youth/sma10-4480

Substance Abuse and Mental Health Services Administration. (2016, August). *Preventing and responding to suicide clusters in American Indian and Alaska native communities report | samhsa library,* Retrieved (May 29, 2026) from https://library.samhsa.gov/product/preventing-and-responding-suicide-clusters-american-indian-and-alaska-native-communities

Substance Abuse and Mental Health Services Administration. (2023a, April 24). *What is mental health?*. SAMHSA, Retrieved (January 31, 2024) from https://www.samhsa.gov/mental-health

Substance Abuse and Mental Health Services Administration. (2023b, June 9). *Samhsa's national helpline*. SAMHSA, Retrieved (January 31, 2024) from https://www.samhsa.gov/find-help/national-helpline

Substance Abuse Mental Health Services Administration. (2023c, April 24). *Help prevent suicide*. SAMHSA, Retrieved (January 31, 2024) from https://www.samhsa.gov/suicide

Substance Abuse Mental Health Services Administration. (2025, July 29). *About suicide and suicidal behavior*, SAMHSA, Retrieved (May 29, 2026) from https://www.samhsa.gov/mental-health/suicidal-behavior/about

Sykes, C., Sweezy, M., Burris, C., Schwartz, R. C., Herbine-Blank, T., Gell, L., McConnell, S., Anderson, F. G., Seligman, C., LaCroix, M., Johnson, S., Locke, K. A., Davidheiser, A., & Pastor, M. (2023, December 21). *What Is Internal Family Systems?*. What is Internal Family Systems?® | IFS Institute, Retrieved (January 31, 2024) from https://ifs-institute.com/

USAFacts. (2023, November 29.-b). USAFACTS. *The US suicide rate has climbed 36% over the past two decades*. USAFacts, Retrieved (January 31, 2024) from https://usafacts.org/articles/how-is-the-suicide-rate-changing-in-the-us/#:~:text=Wyoming%20had%20the%20highest%20state,7.1,%207.9,%20and%208.0.

Wikimedia Foundation. (2024a, January 12). *List of suicide crisis lines*. Wikipedia, Retrieved (January 31, 2024) from https://en.wikipedia.org/wiki/List_of_suicide_crisis_lines

Wikimedia Foundation. (2024b, January 23). *Introduction to quantum mechanics*. Wikipedia. YouTube. Retrieved (January 31, 2024) from https://en.wikipedia.org/wiki/Introduction_to_quantum_mechanics

YouTube. (2017, June 1). *Daily Qigong routine*. YouTube. https://www.youtube.com/watch?v=nmmNWj9YtAw

YouTube. (2023, October 3). *"Pain free" Pete egoscue menu for necks cervical spine / neck herniation cert. by Egoscue Institute.* YouTube, Retrieved (February 2, 2024) from https://www.youtube.com/watch?v=0OpKqPgtXIg

www.ingramcontent.com/pod-product-compliance
Lightning Source LLC
LaVergne TN
LVHW100332210926
848480LV00003B/1311